101

Developmental Concepts & Workouts for Cross Country Runners

Jason R. Karp, Ph.D.

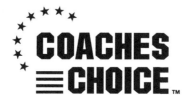

ISBN: 978-1-60679-116-5
Library of Congress Control Number: 2010930065
Cover design: Brenden Murphy
Book layout: Studio J Art & Design
Front cover photo: Sacramento Bee/Randall Benton/ZUMA Press
Illustrations: Hemera/Thinkstock

Coaches Choice
P.O. Box 1828
Monterey, CA 93942
www.coacheschoice.com

Dedication

This book is dedicated to cross country runners around the country,
who pour their hearts into every race they run.

Acknowledgments

I'd like to thank James Peterson of Coaches Choice, who asked me to write this book; the editorial staff at Coaches Choice; my wonderful agent, Grace Freedson; runners Pedro Molina, John Romais, Kim Mueller, and Molly Kline, who served as models for the photographs; my mother, Muriel, for constantly telling me how proud she is of me; and my twin brother, Jack, for accepting that there are two writers in the family.

Introduction

From my very first cross country race as a freshman in high school, I knew that cross country running is a unique sport. The crispness of the autumn air, the morning dew on the grass, the colored leaves at the start of the season and the leaves on the ground by the season's end, uphills, downhills, the starting line of 200 runners anxiously awaiting the starter's gun, the crackling of the 200 pairs of spikes on patches of gravel and pavement between fields of grass and dirt trails, and one winner at the end of the race; there's nothing quite like it. Sigmund Freud once remarked that pure happiness is when you take your foot out from beneath the covers in the middle of winter and then place it back in. To the cross country runner, pure happiness is the exact opposite— when you take your foot out from beneath the covers and leave it out, risking what's uncomfortable. For the cross country runner, pure happiness is not found in satisfying comfort; it is found in dealing with discomfort.

Cross country running began in England in the early 19th century with a game called Hares and Hounds. In this game, a runner or group of runners (the hares) would lay a "scent" by scattering pieces of paper while following a random course, and a second set of runners (the hounds) would then set out in pursuit, trying to follow the paper trail. In 1878, the sport was introduced to the United States as a way to train for summer track and field. Harvard was the first university to incorporate cross country running, with other schools soon following. In 1890, the first intercollegiate meet was held between City College of New York, Cornell University, and the University of Pennsylvania. Cross country runners are often referred to as "harriers," referring to the breed of dog belonging to the hound class.

To train harriers most effectively, *101 Developmental Concepts & Workouts for Cross Country Runners* is divided into two parts. Part 1 presents 30 training concepts to help guide the cross country runner and coach. These concepts lay the groundwork for the 71 workouts included in Part 2, which include variations and coaching points where appropriate. Each workout should be preceded by an adequate warm-up and followed by a cool-down, with the warm-up starting slowly and getting progressively faster until the pace matches the pace that will be used in the workout.

It is my hope that the concepts and workouts presented in this book will help coaches train cross country runners to become faster and more accomplished.

Contents

Concept #1:   To run fast, athletes must first spend a lot of time
running slow.

Concept #2:   Easy runs must be easy.

Concept #3:   Time is more important than miles.

Concept #4:   The three main physiological determinants of distance running
performance are $\dot{V}O_2max$, lactate (acidosis) threshold, and
running economy.

Concept #5:   The lungs do not limit running performance.

Concept #6:   Eating immediately following a workout speeds recovery.

Concept #7:   Only increase the speed of workouts when the athletes'
races have shown that they have achieved a higher level of fitness.

Concept #8:   The goal of training is to use the least stressful stimulus
to cause the desired adaptation.

Concept #9:   Athletes have different muscle-fiber types that will reflect
their strengths and weaknesses and influence their adaptive
responses to training.

Concept #10: Athletes should always be trained to their strengths.

Concept #11: The aim of training is to introduce training stimuli in such
a fashion that higher and higher levels of adaptation are achieved.

Concept #12: The human body is great at adapting to stress *as long as that
stress is applied in small doses.*

Concept #13: If athletes want to improve their performances, their training
load must increase.

Concept #14: Every workout should have a specific purpose.

Concept #15: Recovery is just as important as training.

Concept #16: It is harder to improve fitness than it is to maintain fitness.

Concept #17: Runners lose fitness faster than it is gained.

Concept #18: Variation of training is key.

Concept #19: A long-term, systematic approach to training will yield the best and most consistent results.

Concept #20: Metabolism is tightly regulated by enzymes and oxygen.

Concept #21: There are identifiable predictors of injury.

Concept #22: The recovery intervals of an interval workout are just as important as the work periods.

Concept #23: Heart rate is a great objective measure of training intensity.

Concept #24: Training must be specific to the task.

Concept #25: Athletes compete the way they practice.

Concept #26: Runners adapt to training by responding to signals.

Concept #27: The ability to adapt to a training stimulus decreases with higher levels of training and does not keep occurring indefinitely.

Concept #28: Weight training should never be performed at the expense of running training.

Concept #29: Athletes should run the first half to two-thirds of a race with their heads and the last third to half with their hearts.

Concept #30: Every athlete is an individual.

PART 1

CROSS COUNTRY RUNNING CONCEPTS

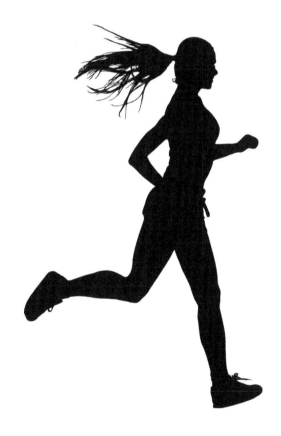

1

Developmental Training Concepts

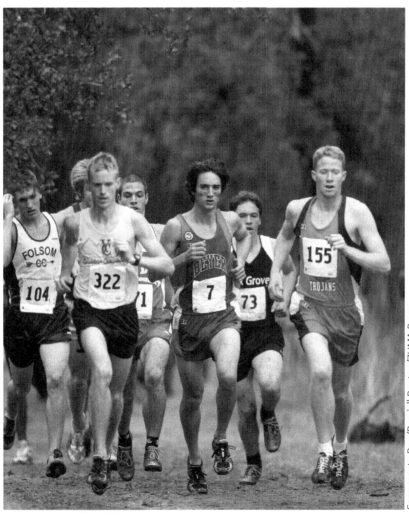

Sacramento Bee/Randall Benton/ZUMA Press

Concept #1: To run fast, athletes must first spend a lot of time running slow.

Although this concept may seem counterintuitive, it is first and foremost the volume of training the cross country runner performs that induces the biological signal for adaptation and dictates the performance capacity. In order to accomplish a large training volume, the runner must perform most of the running at a relatively slow pace. Lots of easy, aerobic running forms the basis of any distance runner's training program. Aerobic running develops many physiological and biochemical traits needed for good endurance. For example, it increases the number of red blood cells and the amount of hemoglobin contained within them, giving athletes' blood vessels a greater oxygen-carrying capability. It also increases muscle capillary volume, providing more oxygen to athletes' muscles. Finally, it increases the volume of mitochondria (the aerobic factories inside muscles) and the number of aerobic enzymes, enabling the muscles to use more oxygen.

Initially, running slow is a difficult concept for young runners to understand. They will likely ask questions like, "Don't I have to run fast in practice to run faster in a race?" and "When are we going to do more speedwork?" While speedwork gives athletes more bang for their buck and improves their performance more quickly than simply running lots of miles, any short-term success may likely occur to the detriment of their long-term development and consistency of performances. The more runners attend to the qualities of aerobic metabolism, the more they will ultimately get from their subsequent speedwork. Since recovery is an aerobic process, being more aerobically fit allows athletes to recover more quickly both during the rest periods of their interval workouts and following a workout. Recovering more quickly within a workout allows athletes to run more repetitions. Since one of the keys to improving VO_2max is to spend as much time as possible running at VO_2max, the benefit to being able to run five 1,000-meter repeats compared to three is obvious. The rapidity with which athletes recover from intense workouts will dictate how often they can perform other intense workouts, which may ultimately influence their ability to reach their running potential.

So, how much aerobic work is enough? It depends on a number of factors, including the athletes' genetically-determined propensity to continually adapt to high mileage and tempo runs, the amount of time they have to run, and the specific racing distance for which they are training. Obviously, the longer the race, the more mileage they need to meet their potential. The best way to determine how much aerobic work each runner needs is to slowly and systematically increase each runner's mileage from month to month and year to year, taking care to note how the runner responds to the training stimulus. Don't increase the mileage unless the prior training and racing experience gives you reason to believe that the runner will continue to improve with more mileage. If the runner hasn't reached a plateau in performance at 40 miles per week, there's no reason yet to increase the mileage to 50.

Concept #2: Easy runs must be easy.

The single-biggest mistake competitive runners make is running too fast on their easy days. By doing so, they add unnecessary stress to their legs without any extra benefit, and they won't be able to run as much quality on their harder days. Speed-type runners (runners who fare better at shorter races) will have a greater difference between their race pace and easy running pace compared to endurance-type runners (runners who fare better at longer races). Since many of the cellular adaptations associated with aerobic training are volume-dependent, not intensity-dependent, the speed of easy runs is not as important as their duration. Slowing down the easy runs has at least three benefits: it decreases the chance of injury, it allows runners to get more out of their harder days because there will be less residual fatigue, and it allows runners to increase their overall weekly mileage. Remember that it is the volume of aerobic running, not the speed, that represents the major stimulus for adaptation. If athletes have heart-rate monitors, aerobic runs should be run at 70 to 75 percent of maximum heart rate.

Concept #3: Time is more important than miles.

Although most runners and coaches think in terms of number of miles run, the amount of time spent running is more important than the number of miles since it's the duration of effort (time spent running) that the runner's body senses. Endurance is improved not by running a specific distance, but by running for a specific amount of time. The duration of effort is one of the key factors that arouse the biological signal to elicit adaptations that will ultimately lead to improvements in running performance. A faster runner will cover the same amount of distance in less time than a slower runner or, to put it another way, will cover more miles in the same amount of time. For example, a runner who averages 7-minute mile pace for 40 miles per week is running the same amount of time as a runner who averages 9-minute mile pace for 31 miles per week (280 minutes per week), and therefore is experiencing the same amount of stress. And that's what matters: the stress. The slower runner may be running fewer miles, but the time spent running—and therefore the stimulus for adaptation—is the same. If a slower runner tries to run as much as a faster runner, the slower runner will experience more stress and therefore put himself at a greater risk for injury. So, at least initially in the training program, the focus should be on time spent running rather than on distance.

Concept #4: The three main physiological determinants of distance running performance are $\dot{V}O_2$max, lactate (acidosis) threshold, and running economy.

$\dot{V}O_2$max is the maximum volume of oxygen your muscles can consume per minute. It is therefore referred to as *aerobic power* since it's a measure of the *rate* at which oxygen is consumed. $\dot{V}O_2$max is considered to be the best single indicator of a person's aerobic fitness. It is determined by both central factors (cardiac output and blood flow to the muscles) and peripheral factors (oxygen extraction and use by the muscles). Mathematically, $\dot{V}O_2$ is equal to the product of the central and peripheral factors: $\dot{V}O_2 = SV \times HR \times$ (a-v O_2 difference), where "SV" is stroke volume (the volume of blood pumped by the heart per beat), "HR" is heart rate, and "a-v O_2 difference" is the difference in oxygen content between arterial blood (the oxygen-rich blood traveling to the muscles) and venous blood (the oxygen-poor blood returning from the muscles to the heart). $\dot{V}O_2$max occurs when SV, HR, and the a-v O_2 difference are all at their maximum values.

The lactate threshold, or what I call the acidosis threshold (AT) because the physiological marker of interest is the acidosis rather than the lactate, demarcates the transition between running that is almost purely aerobic and running that includes significant anaerobic metabolism. (All running speeds have an anaerobic contribution, although when running slower than AT pace, that contribution is negligible.) Thus, the AT is an important determinant of distance running performance since it represents the fastest speed runners can sustain aerobically without a significant anaerobic contribution.

Running economy is the volume of oxygen ($\dot{V}O_2$) used to maintain a given sub-maximum speed. The less oxygen a runner uses to run at a specific speed, the better. For example, if two runners have the same $\dot{V}O_2$max, but Runner A uses 70 percent and Runner B uses 80 percent of that $\dot{V}O_2$max while running at an 8-minute mile pace, the pace feels easier for Runner A because Runner A is more economical. Therefore, Runner A can run at a faster pace before feeling the same amount of fatigue as Runner B.

While $\dot{V}O_2$max has received most of the attention among runners and coaches, and is arguably the most popular of the three determinants of distance running, a high $\dot{V}O_2$max alone is not enough to attain elite-level performances; it simply gives a runner access into the club, since a runner cannot attain a high level of performance without a high $\dot{V}O_2$max. Furthermore, while runners can improve their $\dot{V}O_2$max, it is largely genetically determined and is actually a rather stable parameter of aerobic fitness once the runner is already trained. The other two major physiological determinants of distance running performance—acidosis threshold (AT) and running economy—exert a greater influence on a runner's performance and are more responsive to training. I have tested many athletes in the laboratory with an elite-level $\dot{V}O_2$max, but few of them were capable of running at the elite or even sub-elite level because they did not have a high AT or were not very economical.

Specific workouts to improve AT and $\dot{V}O_2$max appear in Chapters 3 and 4, respectively. Despite its importance, running economy seems to be the most difficult of the three physiological determinants to target with training. However, research has shown that runners who perform high volumes of endurance training tend to be more economical, and that power training—either with heavy weights or plyometric exercises—improves running economy. It is possible that, just as repetition of the walking movement decreases the jerkiness of a toddler's walk to the point that it becomes smooth, repetition of the movements of running (as occurs with high mileage) has an underrecognized neural component. With countless repetitions, motor-unit (muscle-fiber) recruitment patterns, all of the steps involved in muscle contraction, and possibly even the relationship between breathing and limb movement are optimized to minimize the oxygen cost and improve economy. Additionally, economy may be improved by the weight loss that usually accompanies high mileage, which leads to a lower oxygen cost. Power training improves running economy likely by a neural mechanism, as muscles are trained to increase their rate of force development.

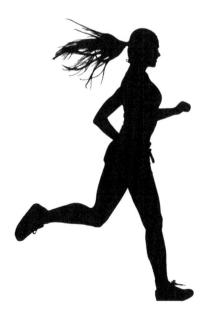

Concept #5: The lungs do not limit running performance.

At first glance, distance running seems to have everything to do with big, strong lungs. After all, it is through the lungs that people get oxygen. If the size of the lungs mattered, you would expect the best distance runners to have large lungs that can hold a lot of oxygen. However, the best distance runners in the world are quite small people, with characteristically small lungs. Total lung capacity, the maximal amount of air the lungs can hold, is primarily influenced by body size, with bigger people having larger lung capacities. Research has shown that the lungs do not limit a runner's ability, especially if the runner is not elite. That limitation rests on the shoulders of the runner's cardiovascular and metabolic systems, with blood flow to and oxygen use by the muscles the major culprits. No relationship exists between lung capacity and how fast someone runs a 5K.

Unlike the cardiovascular and muscular systems, research suggests that the pulmonary system does not adapt to training. Therefore, the lungs may only limit performance in elite runners who have developed the more trainable characteristics of aerobic metabolism (e.g., cardiac output, hemoglobin concentration, and mitochondrial and capillary volumes) to capacities that approach the genetic potential of the lungs to provide for adequate diffusion of oxygen. In other words, the lungs may limit performance in elite runners by "lagging behind" other, more readily adaptable characteristics. But this is only a problem when those other characteristics have been trained enough to reach their genetic potential.

Humans' main stimulus to breathe (at sea level) is an increase in the blood's carbon dioxide content. Athletes breathe more during faster-paced workouts and races not because they need more oxygen, but because more carbon dioxide is being produced in their muscles and needs to be expelled through the lungs. Oxygen is all around and has no problem diffusing from the air into the lungs. What is important in the lungs, however, is the process of oxygen diffusion from the alveoli of the lungs into the pulmonary capillaries. The pulmonary capillaries feed into the left side of the heart, which is responsible for pumping blood and oxygen to the runner's organs, including the muscles used to run. This elegant process of diffusion is already more than adequate, even when running at racing speeds—at sea level, the hemoglobin in the runner's blood is nearly 100 percent saturated with oxygen, both at rest and even while running a race. (In some elite runners, whose hearts pump large quantities of blood through the lungs each minute, the hemoglobin in their blood becomes desaturated of oxygen when running at race pace, a condition called "exercise-induced hypoxemia.") The situation is slightly different at higher altitudes, where athletes breathe more to compensate for their blood being less saturated with oxygen.

Since the blood is already nearly maximally saturated with oxygen, it's fruitless to take deeper breaths in an attempt to get in more oxygen, as many runners try to do. Furthermore, the extra muscle action of the diaphragm and other breathing muscles necessary for a larger inspiration may take away some of the oxygen needed by the leg muscles. During moderate running, the oxygen cost of breathing is approximately 3 to 6 percent of total body oxygen consumption ($\dot{V}O_2$max), while during maximal running, it is about 10 percent of $\dot{V}O_2$max, costing as much as 13 to 15 percent in some athletes. Since runners increase oxygen delivery to their muscles by increasing both heart rate and stroke volume, they should focus on methods to increase maximum stroke volume rather than taking deeper breaths.

Concept #6: Eating immediately following a workout speeds recovery.

It's easy for high school and even college athletes to not eat after a workout. But not refueling after they run is possibly the single worst thing they can do to thwart their recovery. Research has shown that delaying carbohydrate ingestion for just two hours after a workout can significantly reduce the rate at which glycogen (the stored form of carbohydrates) is synthesized and stored in the muscles and liver.

Refueling after workouts is important for several reasons, including the replenishment of fuel stores and the repair of cellular damage. In regards to fuel, carbohydrates are the most important nutrient to replenish after a workout. Endurance performance is strongly influenced by the amount of pre-exercise muscle glycogen, with intense endurance exercise decreasing muscle glycogen content. Glycogen synthesis is a complex biochemical process largely controlled by the hormone insulin and the availability and uptake of glucose from the circulation. To maximize the rate of glycogen synthesis, athletes should consume 0.7 gram of simple carbohydrates (sugar, preferably glucose) per pound of body weight within 30 minutes after they run and every two hours for four to six hours.

Regarding reparation of cellular damage, protein is another important nutrient to consume after hard and long runs. To repair muscle fibers that are damaged during training, athletes should consume 20 to 30 grams of complete protein (those which contain all essential amino acids) after they run.

Since nutrients in fluids are absorbed more quickly than from solid foods, athletes should initially consume carbohydrates in a drink. Despite the many highly advertised commercial sports drinks, any beverage that contains a large amount of carbohydrates will be great for recovery. Chocolate milk, which is high in both carbohydrates and protein, is a great post-workout recovery drink.

Concept #7: Only increase the speed of workouts when the athletes' races have shown that they have achieved a higher level of fitness.

Most runners, especially younger ones, want to push the pace all the time. They want to run their workouts faster because they believe that to run faster in races, they need to run faster in workouts. However, this thinking is backwards. Races tell the coach and the athletes what their current level of fitness is right now. Races dictate the training paces, not the other way around. Runners don't do workouts to practice running faster. They do workouts to improve the physiological characteristics that will allow them to run faster in the future. Think of an assembly line: If you want to make more products, the better strategy is to increase the number of workers (physiological characteristics) so you have more assembly lines to do the work, rather than increase the speed at which the assembly line workers work. To make the workouts more difficult, increase the amount of time (or number of repetitions) that athletes spend at the desired pace or effort rather than having them run faster. When running intervals, workouts can also be made more difficult by decreasing the time of the recovery periods. When athletes run faster races, then adjust the workout paces to agree with the newly achieved level of fitness.

Concept #8: The goal of training is to use the least stressful stimulus to cause the desired adaptation.

Runners often perform workouts at speeds that are too fast to obtain the desired result. The problem is that they don't know what the desired result is. To determine the correct speed, you must know the purpose of each workout. For example, say you want to improve your athletes' $\dot{V}O_2$max, and they plan to run 1,000-meter repeats at the speed at $\dot{V}O_2$max. If running each 1,000-meter repeat in 3:30 elicits $\dot{V}O_2$max during the work period (which is the goal of the workout), running each repeat in 3:20 will certainly also elicit $\dot{V}O_2$max. But why run each repeat in 3:20 when they can run it in 3:30 and still get the same benefit? To improve $\dot{V}O_2$max, running faster than $\dot{V}O_2$max pace is not better than running at $\dot{V}O_2$max pace. All running faster does is add more fatigue to the athletes' legs without any extra benefit. For anaerobic capacity workouts, the speed should be just fast enough to cause acidosis and recruit fast-twitch muscle fibers—800-meter to mile race pace for competitive runners. Running at the correct pace will more specifically target the physiological variable you're trying to train.

Concept #9: Athletes have different muscle-fiber types that will reflect their strengths and weaknesses and influence their adaptive responses to training.

There are two types of runners—runners who have superior speed, whose performance gets better as the race gets shorter, and runners who have superior endurance, whose performance gets better as the race gets longer. Much of this difference is due to differences is muscle-fiber composition, which is genetically determined.

Humans have three different types of muscle fibers, with gradations between them. Slow-twitch (ST) fibers are recruited for all aerobic runs, while fast-twitch B (FT-B) fibers are only recruited for short anaerobic, high-force production activities, such as sprinting. Fast-twitch A (FT-A) fibers, which represent a transition between the two extremes of ST and FT-B fibers, are recruited for prolonged anaerobic activities with a relatively high-force output, such as racing 400 meters, and are also recruited when the slow-twitch fibers fatigue. It's a given that cross country runners have more ST fibers than FT fibers, otherwise they would be sprinters rather than distance runners. However, even within a group of distance runners, a disparity is still found in the amount of ST fibers. Some runners may have 90 percent ST and 10 percent FT fibers, while others may have 60 percent ST and 40 percent FT fibers.

Understanding the differences in fiber types between athletes (and thus the athletes' strengths and weaknesses) can help the coach be smarter about training athletes. For example, an endurance-type runner (a runner who has a large proportion of ST fibers) should focus on aerobic work (mileage and acidosis threshold workouts). A speed-type runner (a runner who has a large proportion of FT fibers) should do less aerobic work (but still adequate enough to meet the demands of the race) and emphasize interval training. Since all of the runners on a cross country team are training to race the same distance, the endurance-type runner should initially do longer intervals, trying to get faster with training, such as 1,200-meter repeats at 5K race pace, increasing speed to 3K race pace or decreasing the recovery as training progresses. The speed-type runner should do shorter intervals, trying to hold the pace for longer with training, such as 800-meter repeats at 3K race pace, increasing the distance to 1,200 meters or increasing the number of repeats as training progresses. Thus, two paths can be taken to meet at the same point.

To determine athletes' strengths and weaknesses, ask them the following questions:
- Which condition best describes how you race?
  - (a) You're able to hang with your competitors during the middle stages, but get outkicked in the last quarter- to half-mile.
  - (b) You have a hard time maintaining the pace during the middle stages, but can finish fast and outkick others.

- Which type of workouts feel easier and more natural?
  - (a) Long intervals (800-meter to mile repeats), long runs, and tempo runs
  - (b) Short, fast intervals (200- to 400-meter repeats)
- Which workouts do you look forward to more?
  - (a) Long intervals, long runs, and tempo runs
  - (b) Short, fast intervals

If the athletes choose (a), they are more endurance-type distance runners, likely with a greater proportion of ST muscle fibers; if they choose (b), they are more speed-type distance runners, likely with a greater proportion of FT muscle fibers.

Concept #10: Athletes should always be trained to their strengths.

While improving athletes' weaknesses will make them more successful, focusing on their strengths will ultimately lead to the best result. Therefore, training should always be skewed in favor of what the runner is naturally good at. It's best to target weaknesses in the preseason or early season phases of training and focus on strengths later in the season, as the athlete gets closer to the most important races.

Concept #11: The aim of training is to introduce training stimuli in such a fashion that higher and higher levels of adaptation are achieved.

Following a training stress, the body adapts and physiologically overcompensates so that if the same stress is encountered again, it does not cause the same degree of physiological disruption. In short, the body adapts to be able to handle the stress. Following the adaptation, the runner can do more work.

Think of each workout as a small threat to some aspect of the body's survival. If athletes repeatedly threaten their bodies' survival, they will make adaptations to assuage the threat. For example, repeatedly running at fast speeds that cause acidosis presents a threat to the muscles' survival by creating an environment that inhibits enzyme function, disrupts glycolysis, decreases muscle force production, and causes fatigue. If you cause acidosis, the muscle says, "Hey, this person is running so fast that I'm becoming acidic. I won't be able to survive. If this activity is going to be a regular habit, I need to create a better buffer to defend the acidosis and maintain my acid-base balance." So, guess what happens? Athletes respond to the repeated acidosis by increasing the size of their muscles' pool of bicarbonate ions, as well as making other adaptations, thus increasing their capacity to do more anaerobic work.

Concept #12: The human body is great at adapting to stress *as long as that stress is applied in small doses.*

When the stress is too severe, or not enough recovery has preceded the new stress, athletes can get injured. Therefore, the training must be systematic along with being progressive. The main reason why runners get injured is because they do too much too soon. Therefore, never increase running volume more than 10 to 15 percent per week, never increase intensity more than 5 percent per week, never increase volume and intensity at the same time, and never introduce too many training variables at the same time (e.g., an increase in running mileage, strength training, and plyometrics). Introduce one training variable, give athletes time to adapt to that new variable, then add another variable, give athletes time to adapt to that new variable, then add another variable.

Concept #13: If athletes want to improve their performances, their training load must increase.

When athletes begin a training program, they will experience many signaling responses and subsequent adaptations. However, continual training at the same level decreases the training-specific signaling responses involved in the adaptations to training. In other words, if an athlete's training stays the same, she can expect her performances to stay the same. For example, if an athlete runs 10 miles on Sunday morning when she is used to running only 8, a strong signal will be sent to make specific adaptations (e.g., an increase in mitochondria, muscle glycogen content, etc.). If the athlete continues to run 10 miles every Sunday for a period of time, she will continue to send signals to make adaptations until those adaptations are fully realized. After the athlete has run 10 miles so many times that she has become habituated to it, a 10-mile run will no longer be enough of a stimulus to initiate any further adaptations. Therefore, if the athlete wants to force more adaptations, she must run longer than 10 miles (or run the miles faster). To become a faster runner, an athlete must gradually and systematically increase the amount of stress so that she increases the signaling response and subsequent adaptations.

Concept #14: Every workout should have a specific purpose.

Training is not arbitrary. Every day that athletes attend practice, the coach should know what it is the athletes are trying to accomplish. Each phase of training, each week, and each workout should be designed around a specific purpose. Most often, the purpose is physiological, but it can also be psychological.

Concept #15: Recovery is just as important as training.

Recovery may be the most overlooked aspect of training. Most runners and coaches focus on how many miles and what pace to run. Improvements in fitness, however, occur during the *recovery* period between training sessions, not during the training itself. Positive physiological adaptations to training occur when a correctly timed alternation between stress and recovery is undertaken. When an athlete finishes a workout, he is weaker, not stronger. How much weaker depends on the intensity and duration of the workout. If the stress is too great and/or the athlete doesn't recover before the next workout or race, his performance and his ability to adapt to subsequent training sessions will decline. The faster and more complete the athlete's recovery, the more he will get out of his training and racing. A number of factors affect the rate of recovery, including the athlete's age, with younger runners recovering faster between workouts; sex, with males typically recovering faster than females; environment, with altitude and cold weather slowing recovery; training intensity, with higher intensity workouts requiring longer recovery time; psychological factors, with stress slowing recovery; nutrition, with a lack of nutrients slowing recovery; and level of cardiovascular fitness, with a high level of cardiovascular fitness speeding recovery due to the quicker delivery of nutrients and removal of metabolic waste by the circulatory system. While much of training is science, manipulating stress and recovery in an organized and systematic training program to get the greatest adaptation possible is an art and needs to be practiced and fine-tuned like other forms of art.

Concept #16: It is harder to improve fitness than it is to maintain fitness.

Unfortunately, improvements in fitness are achieved somewhat slowly because cellular changes are occurring. However, once an athlete has achieved a high level of fitness, maintaining that fitness level is easier than what it took to achieve that level of fitness in the first place. To maintain fitness, the intensity of training is more important than either the volume (i.e., weekly mileage) or the frequency (i.e., number of days per week). As long as runners keep the intensity high, they can maintain their fitness level.

Concept #17: Runners lose fitness faster than it is gained.

Anyone who has ever been injured and has been forced to take time off from running knows how quickly fitness is lost. A lot of truth is found in the old adage: "Use it, or lose it." With the consistent introduction of training stimuli, constant signals are sent to create adaptations. Those adaptations occur to assuage the threats that have been imposed. Once the stimuli are removed, not only are signals no longer sent to create any further adaptations, there is no longer any reason to keep the adaptations that have occurred. So, the body gets rid of them, which is why it is so important to prevent athletes from becoming injured—because they will not only lose the time off due to the injury, they will also have a very long road back to regain the fitness that was lost during the break.

Concept #18: Variation of training is key.

Research has shown that training programs with variation have more benefit than those with no variation. When a new stress is introduced, athletes need some time to adapt to the new stress. Given enough time, however, the athletes will habituate to the stress. Therefore, once the adaptations to the stress are realized, athletes should change the stimulus. Since cross country runners need to improve many types of fitness—including aerobic fitness, anaerobic fitness, muscular endurance, muscular power, and speed— varying the training stimuli is integral to their success.

Concept #19: A long-term, systematic approach to training will yield the best and most consistent results.

Training is not like cooking, simply mixing ingredients together in a skillet and adding a little salt and pepper. It is much more planned and systematic; nothing is done for the sheer sake of variety. Every month and every year of training should build on what came before it, with each year creating a larger aerobic base to lift the athlete's level of performance to a higher peak.

Concept #20: Metabolism is tightly regulated by enzymes and oxygen.

Enzymes function as biological catalysts that speed up chemical reactions. In the absence of enzymes, chemical reactions would not occur quickly enough to generate the energy needed to run. The amount of an enzyme also controls which metabolic pathway is used. For example, having more aerobic enzymes will steer metabolism toward a greater reliance on aerobic metabolism at a given sub-maximum speed. Enzymes are also activated or inhibited (i.e., their effectiveness in speeding up chemical reactions can be either increased or decreased), determining which metabolic pathways are functional during certain cellular conditions. Thus, enzymes essentially control metabolism and therefore control the pace at which runners fatigue. The link between an increase in mitochondrial enzyme activity and an increase in mitochondria's capacity to consume oxygen, first made in 1967 in the muscles of rats, has provided much insight into the adaptability of skeletal muscle with training. Research has shown that both aerobic and anaerobic training increase enzyme activity.

Metabolism is also regulated by its patriarch—oxygen. The availability of oxygen determines which metabolic pathway predominates. For example, at the end of the metabolic pathway that breaks down carbohydrates (glycolysis), there is a fork in the road. When there is enough oxygen available to meet the muscle's needs, the final product of glycolysis—pyruvate—is converted into an important metabolic intermediate that enters the Krebs cycle for oxidation. This irreversible conversion of pyruvate inside muscles' mitochondria is a decisive reaction in metabolism since it commits the carbohydrates broken down through glycolysis to be oxidized by the Krebs cycle. However, when there is not enough oxygen available to meet the muscle's needs, pyruvate is converted into lactate. An associated consequence of this latter fate is the accumulation of metabolites and the development of acidosis, causing muscles to fatigue and the athlete to slow down.

The more aerobically developed cross country runners are, by focusing on increasing their mileage and doing AT workouts, the more they'll steer pyruvate toward the Krebs cycle and away from lactate production at a given pace. That's a good thing, because the amount of energy runners get from pyruvate entering the Krebs cycle is 19 times greater than what they get from pyruvate being converted into lactate. While pyruvate will always be converted into lactate given a fast enough speed, the goal of training is to increase the speed at which that occurs.

Concept #21: There are identifiable predictors of injury.

While sometimes athletes get injured without any apparent reason and no matter how careful the coach, a number of factors can predict the likelihood of an athlete getting injured. The problem is that coaches don't often take the time or make the effort to identify them. Many injuries can be prevented if athletes are screened for the following risk factors.

Low Energy Availability

Given the large number of calories expended from many miles of running, athletes need to make sure that they consume enough calories to offset their high caloric expenditure. Many athletes simply don't eat enough to meet their needs for specific nutrients, like calcium and vitamin D, which can put their bones at risk for injury. Low energy availability is a key risk factor for stress fractures, especially among female runners. Athletes need to consume 1,000 milligrams of calcium per day and 400 International Units of vitamin D per day.

Female Athlete Triad

The largest risk for stress fractures in female runners occurs when they have one or more of three associated characteristics—menstrual irregularities, disordered eating, and osteoporosis—collectively called the female athlete triad. High training volumes can cause irregular or even absent menstrual cycles (amenorrhea), which increase the risk for osteoporosis and stress fractures. Research has shown that female athletes with irregular menstruation or amenorrhea have a lower bone mineral density than female athletes with normal menstruation. Disordered eating (not to be confused with an eating disorder, like anorexia or bulimia), common among female athletes due to external or self-imposed pressure to lose weight, may result in caloric restriction, and is independently associated with both irregular menstruation and low bone mineral density. In other words, an athlete could have normal menstruation and still have low bone mineral density if her dietary habits are inadequate to meet her caloric needs. Athletes who have any of the characteristics of the female athlete triad should regularly have their bone mineral density assessed to determine if they are at risk for injury. If they do have low bone mineral density, they may want to take birth-control pills, which provide their bodies with bone-protecting estrogen.

Previous Injury

Athletes who have had an injury are at an increased risk for another one. Already having an injury shows that body part is vulnerable.

Large Increases in Training Load

The majority of injuries, including tendonitis and stress fractures, result from doing too much too soon. For example, the common injury of shin splints (medial tibial stress syndrome), which occurs most often in newer and younger runners, is typically caused by exposure to excessive shock to which the bone is initially unable to adapt. To prevent large increases in training load, athletes should increase the length and intensity of their runs by no more than 10 to 15 percent per week and back off on the volume for one week every few weeks to allow their bodies to adapt to the training, recover from the training stress, and stay injury-free. Not only must the coach be meticulous and careful in designing the training program, the coach must also know exactly what the athletes have been doing, especially during breaks from school. Too often, athletes get injured in the beginning of the season because they jump into the coach's fall training plan, not having followed the plan the coach set for them during the summer. It's also easy for athletes to get re-injured when they return to training after being injured because it's easy to just jump right into what everyone else on the team is doing.

Strength Imbalances

Muscle strength imbalances, like those between the quadriceps and the hamstrings and between the calves and the muscles on the front of the shin can lead to muscle and tendon injuries. Athletes should attend to these imbalances by strengthening their weaker muscles.

Lack of Running Experience

Runners who lack experience (e.g., high school underclassmen) are at a great risk for injuries. Therefore, extra care must be taken when increasing the volume and intensity of inexperienced runners' training. Inexperienced runners may need to spend a few weeks at the same training load before increasing the load.

Inappropriate Running Shoes

Running shoes must be appropriate for the athlete's foot type and running mechanics. Running shoes have specific combinations of support and stability designed for different running gaits. Cushioning shoes, which are best suited for runners with normal to high arches, promote adequate pronation to absorb shock upon landing. Stability shoes, which are best suited for runners with normal to low arches and who slightly overpronate, allow only limited pronation and retain some cushioning characteristics. Motion-control shoes, which are best suited for runners with flat feet and who severely overpronate, prevent pronation. Running in the wrong shoes can adversely affect lower extremity alignment, making runners more susceptible to injury. For example, predisposing factors for Achilles tendonitis include a shoe that twists easily, insufficient heel height, and a rigid sole. Running shoes should be replaced after 300 to 400 miles because they lose their shock-absorbing abilities.

Concept #22: The recovery intervals of an interval workout are just as important as the work periods.

While the focus of interval workouts is almost always on the work periods—how fast, how long, how many repetitions—the reason they are called "interval workouts" or "intervals" is because of the recovery interval between work periods. When interval training was first studied in the 1950s, the belief was that the primary stimulus for cardiovascular improvement occurs not during the period of activity, but during the recovery interval. The original interval training method incorporated periods of effort ranging from 30 to 70 seconds at an intensity that elevated the heart rate to about 180 beats per minute. The effort phase was followed by sufficient recovery time to allow the heart rate to return to 120 beats per minute, signifying the readiness to perform the next work period.

During the recovery interval, the heart rate declines at a proportionally greater rate than the return of blood to the heart, resulting in a brief increase in stroke volume (the amount of blood the heart pumps with each beat). The increase in stroke volume places an overload on the heart muscle, which makes the heart stronger, and enables the skeletal muscles to be cleared of waste products quickly due to the elevated rate of blood flow when there is little demand for activity from the tissues. Since stroke volume peaks during the recovery interval, and because there are many recovery intervals during an interval workout, stroke volume peaks many times, providing a stimulus for improving maximum stroke volume and thus the capacity of the oxygen transport system.

Also during the recovery intervals, a portion of the muscular stores of runners' quick energy—adenosine triphosphate (ATP) and creatine phosphate (CP)—that were depleted during the preceding work period is replenished via the aerobic system. During each work period that follows a recovery period, the replenished ATP and CP will again be available as an energy source.

While it may be more difficult to monitor heart rates during the recovery intervals if athletes don't have heart-rate monitors, they can determine their heart rate the old-fashioned way by palpating either their carotid or radial artery and counting pulses for 10 seconds and multiplying by 6.

Concept #23: Heart rate is a great objective measure of training intensity.

A positive linear relationship is found between running intensity and heart rate—as intensity increases, so does heart rate. Thus, athletes can use heart rate to train at specific intensities. For example, during easy runs, heart rate can be used to ensure the intensity remains low so that athletes sufficiently recover from the previous day's workout. During interval workouts, heart rate can be used to ensure the intensity is high enough to get the most cardiovascular bang for the buck. Heart rate can also be used to monitor athletes' progress over time. For example, as athletes' fitness improves, they will be running at a faster pace when at the same heart rate or, to put it another way, their heart rate will be lower when running at the same pace. As a guide, the following are heart rate values for specific workouts:

- Easy runs: 70 to 75 percent max heart rate
- Lactate (Acidosis) threshold runs: 85 to 90 percent max heart rate
- $\dot{V}O_2$max intervals: 95 to 100 percent max heart rate

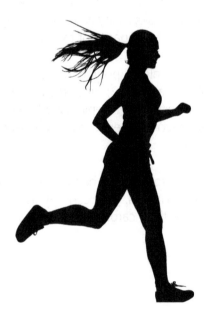

Concept #24: Training must be specific to the task.

Functional changes take place only in the organs, cells, and intracellular structures that are stressed during physical activity. If athletes want bigger biceps, doing squats won't help. Muscles adapt to the specific demands placed on them. In addition to the physiological changes that take place inside athletes' muscles, training also involves a motor-unit (muscle-fiber) recruitment aspect. The brain needs to learn to communicate with the muscles to perform a specific task, and the muscles need to learn to produce force at specific joint angles and against specific surfaces, which influence the amount of force muscles can produce. Therefore, athletes need to train the entire movement pattern, rather than the strength or endurance of individual muscles or single-joint movements. That's why someone has to run to be a good runner and ride a bike to be a good cyclist. Running won't help you become a better cyclist any more than riding a bike will help you become a better runner. The movement patterns of the two activities are completely different and therefore differ in their motor-unit recruitment patterns and their muscles' ability to produce force. To become accomplished at an activity, athletes must practice that activity and not expect to improve their performance by doing some other activity.

Cross country runners need to accustom their muscles and tendons to cross country terrain by running as much as they can on cross country courses that include grass and dirt. This includes all formal workouts as well, like tempo runs and intervals, and even when the weather is bad and the ground is wet. Good runners will run well regardless of the terrain, but doing workouts on a track to prepare for a cross country race is like a tennis player practicing on a hard court to prepare for a tournament on a clay or grass court. The way a tennis player's feet move and the way the ball bounces on a clay or grass court are different from on a hard court, just like running on a track is different from running on grass fields and dirt trails, where they experience more side-to-side ankle movement. Athletes need to train on the surface they plan to race. Therefore, all of the workouts presented in this book should be done on cross country courses.

Concept #25: Athletes compete the way they practice.

While this concept is not specific only to cross country running, it should be mentioned here since athletes will race the way they train. For example, athletes who always start a tempo run or an interval workout too fast and get slower with each successive mile or repetition will likely also run a race like that. Athletes must practice how to race.

Concept #26: Runners adapt to training by responding to signals.

How much runners adapt to a training stimulus ultimately depends on how responsive their cells are to signals. Muscle cells are able to detect all kinds of signals—mechanical, metabolic, neural, and hormonal, which are amplified and transmitted via signaling cascades and lead to the events involved in gene expression. This signaling is fast, occurring within minutes of completing a workout. Signaling results in the activation of transcription factors, which are proteins that bind to a specific part of DNA and control the transfer of genetic information from DNA to RNA.

Many of the physiological and biochemical adaptations to training begin with the runner's DNA, with the copying of one of its double helical strands (a process called replication). The replicated DNA strand, under the action of transcription factors, is then transcribed into messenger RNA (a process called transcription), and the messenger RNA is then translated into a protein (a process called translation). Finally, the protein is transported from the nucleus of the cell where transcription and translation occur to the place where it will function.

While a single workout alone, especially if it is new to the athlete, introduces a specific signal and activation of transcription factors, repeated workouts lead to a concerted accumulation of messenger RNAs that can be translated into a host of structural and functional proteins. In the case of distance running, the accumulation of proteins is manifested, for example, as an increase in the number of mitochondria, the microscopic aerobic factories responsible for aerobic metabolism.

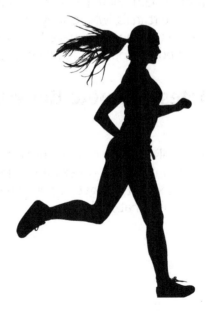

Concept #27: The ability to adapt to a training stimulus decreases with higher levels of training and does not keep occurring indefinitely.

A point will come, which is specific to each runner, when more training does not lead to more adaptations and faster race times. For example, while mitochondrial density is highly modifiable, with the number of mitochondria in skeletal muscle increasing in response to endurance training, there is a threshold above which further increases in training volume do not result in further increases in mitochondrial density. One of the main differences between great runners and good runners is that great runners continue to make physiological adaptations with more and more training. When a young runner is untrained, improvements in performance come quickly, even with modest training. For example, a young runner who doubles her training volume from 20 miles per week to 40 miles per week will likely see a large improvement in performance. However, as more and more training is undertaken, the return on the investment becomes smaller and smaller. The better a runner gets, the harder it is to improve, despite a lot more training. For example, if an athlete is running 50 miles per week and increases training volume by 50 percent to 75 miles per week, her performance will not improve by 50 percent. (That would be the equivalent of improving from an 18-minute 5K to a 9-minute 5K!) One of the goals of training, assuming the athlete is motivated enough to realize her capabilities, is to find out where that "point of no return" is. As training load continues to increase, a point will come when the return on investment is smaller than the risk of injury. In this case, the coach must decide whether the possible small improvement in performance is worth the injury risk.

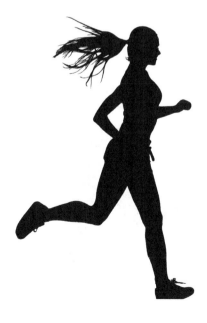

Concept #28: Weight training should never be performed at the expense of running training.

Despite all of the attention given to weight training among athletes and coaches, weight training is not necessary for cross country runners unless they have maximized their running training by increasing both mileage and intensity, cannot handle the physical stress of running more miles, and/or have reached their genetic limit for adaptation to the running training. Like other endurance sports, cross country running is primarily limited by the delivery and use of oxygen. No studies show that weight training improves oxygen delivery from lungs to muscles, which is largely dictated by the athlete's cardiac output (the amount of blood pumped by the heart per minute), the amount of red blood cells and hemoglobin in the athlete's blood, and the athlete's muscles' capillary and mitochondrial volumes.

While weight training, especially when performed to increase muscle power production, may be beneficial, most runners are better served by spending more time running and improving the cardiovascular and metabolic parameters associated with endurance than by weight training. For most runners, it's better to increase running volume from 30 to 40 miles per week (or from 40 to 50 miles per week) than to remain at 30 miles per week and include weight training. Most athletes have a limited amount of time and energy to devote to training. Given the importance of the specificity of training discussed in Concept #24, most of that available time should be spent performing the activity the athlete wants to master. Having said that, supplemental training, including form drills, core strengthening, and dynamic flexibility exercises, can help athletes tolerate greater running training loads and prevent injuries. See Chapter 10 for supplemental training.

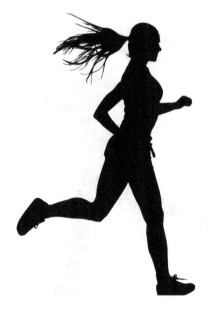

Concept #29: Athletes should run the first half to two-thirds of a race with their heads and the last third to half with their hearts.

Young runners are often emotional at the start of a cross country race, but running with one's emotions in the beginning rarely works in a cross country race. There's a time and a place for emotions and heart, but it's not in the first mile.

Concept #30: Every athlete is an individual.

While this concept may seem obvious, too often it is neglected. There is a large inter-individual response to training, both in the magnitude of response and in the time frame for developing and retaining training effects. What may work for one athlete may not work for another. Not all athletes who are capable of the same performance have the same work capacity. Some athletes may respond better to high volume and low intensity, while some may respond better to low volume and high intensity. Some need more recovery days between hard workouts than others. Therefore, it is important for coaches to know the training needs of their athletes and to individualize their athletes' training while still maintaining a team atmosphere.

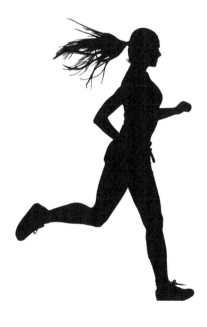

PART 2

CROSS COUNTRY RUNNING WORKOUTS

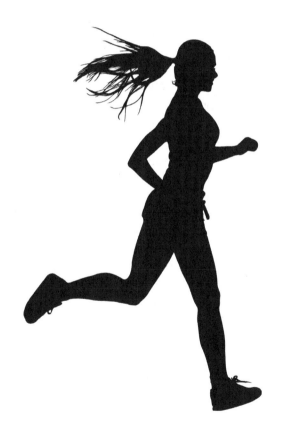

2

Aerobic Training

To provide the energy for muscle contraction, a high-energy chemical compound called adenosine triphosphate (ATP) is broken down into its constituents—adenosine diphosphate (ADP) and inorganic phosphate (P_i). Since muscles don't store much ATP, humans must constantly resynthesize it. The formation and resynthesis of ATP is thus a circular process—ATP is broken down into ADP and P_i, and then ADP and P_i combine to resynthesize ATP. Running faster comes down to increasing the rate at which ATP is resynthesized so it can be broken down to liberate energy for muscle contraction.

For cross country runners, the aerobic system is the predominant energy system used to resynthesize ATP. The rate at which cross country runners can resynthesize ATP for muscle contraction is limited by their aerobic capacity. Therefore, the development of a cross country runner begins with aerobic training, which comprises the majority of a cross country runner's training. Aerobic training stimulates many physiological, biochemical, and molecular adaptations, such as an increase in the number of red blood cells and hemoglobin, which improves blood vessels' oxygen-carrying capability; an increased storage of more fuel (glycogen) in the skeletal muscles; an increased use of intramuscular fat at the same speed to spare glycogen; a greater capillary network for a more rapid diffusion of oxygen into the muscles; and, through the complex activation of gene expression, an increase in mitochondrial density and the number of aerobic enzymes, which increases the muscles' aerobic metabolic capacity. All of these adaptations can be thought of as the body's attempt to cope with the demand placed on it by running every day.

Not only do the majority of improvements in cross country running performance come from increasing aerobic fitness, a high aerobic capacity is beneficial to an athlete doing anaerobic work. An athlete with a well-trained aerobic system will recover faster from the anaerobic training than one who lacks a high level of aerobic fitness.

Workout #1: Short-Distance Run

Objective: To achieve the desired weekly mileage and "fill in" between harder workout days.

Description: Athletes run from 30 to 45 minutes over flat or rolling terrain at an easy pace (about 1 1/2 to 2 minutes per mile slower than 5K race pace). If athletes run twice per day, short-distance runs can be done in the morning.

Coaching Point: This workout is the most common type of workout for cross country runners. Try to vary the place and terrain to keep athletes motivated and inspired.

Workout #2: Medium-Distance Run

Objective: To achieve the desired weekly mileage and add a bit more stress to the normal short-distance run.

Description: Athletes run from 45 to 75 minutes over flat or rolling terrain. This run can be done once per week, preferably in the middle of the week. More accomplished runners may do two medium-distance runs per week.

Coaching Point: Ensure athletes do not do their medium-distance runs too fast.

Workout #3: Long-Distance Run

Objective: To achieve the desired weekly mileage and add a bit more stress to the normal short-distance run.

Description: Athletes run from 75 minutes to two hours over flat or rolling terrain. The long-distance run is done once per week. Lengthen the long run by one mile each week for three or four weeks before backing off (by about a third) for a recovery week.

Coaching Point: Long runs should be significantly longer than any of the other daily runs, but be capped at about 30 percent of the athlete's weekly mileage to prevent injury.

Workout #4: Long Accelerating Run

Objective: To add more quality (and thus more stress) to the normal long-distance run.

Description: This workout is a long run that starts slow and gets progressively faster every few miles. Depending on their ability and typical length of their long runs, athletes run 8 to 15 miles, running the first quarter at an easy pace, the second quarter at slightly slower than acidosis-threshold pace (see Chapter 3 on acidosis (lactate) threshold training), the third quarter at acidosis-threshold pace, and the fourth quarter at faster than acidosis-threshold pace.

Coaching Point: Since this run is pretty demanding, athletes should do the long accelerating run every other week.

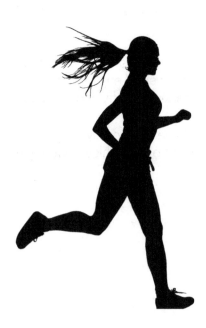

3

Acidosis (Lactate) Threshold Training

The acidosis threshold (AT) demarcates the transition between running that is almost purely aerobic and running that includes significant oxygen-independent (anaerobic) metabolism. (All running speeds have an anaerobic contribution, although when running slower than acidosis-threshold pace, that contribution is negligible.) Therefore, the AT represents the fastest speed that can be sustained aerobically. Research has shown that the AT is the best physiological predictor of distance running performance.

Training the AT increases the speed at which acidosis occurs, enabling athletes to run at a higher percentage of $\dot{V}O_2$max for a longer time. Increasing the AT pace allows runners to run faster before they fatigue because it allows them to run faster before oxygen-independent metabolism begins to play a significant role. What was once an anaerobic pace becomes high aerobic. Imagine two runners who have similar $\dot{V}O_2$max values but differ in their AT paces. If Runner A and Runner B both have a $\dot{V}O_2$max of 60 milliliters of oxygen per kilogram per minute (ml/kg/min), but Runner A's AT is 70 percent and Runner B's AT is 80 percent of $\dot{V}O_2$max, Runner B can sustain a higher intensity and will beat Runner A. Also, a runner with a lower $\dot{V}O_2$max can perform similarly to a runner with a higher $\dot{V}O_2$max if she has a higher AT. If Runner X has a $\dot{V}O_2$max of 50 ml/kg/min and an AT that is 80 percent of her $\dot{V}O_2$max and Runner Y has a $\dot{V}O_2$max of 60 ml/kg/min and an AT that is 67 percent of her $\dot{V}O_2$max, Runner X will be able to sustain a similar intensity as Runner Y, despite having a lower $\dot{V}O_2$max (80 percent of 50 = 40 ml/kg/min vs. 67 percent of 60 = 40 ml/kg/min).

AT workouts are not all-out. They are high-end aerobic. The pace should feel comfortably hard. AT workouts are the most difficult type for athletes to run at the correct speed, especially those runners who are young or inexperienced with these workouts, since these workouts require holding back and not pushing the pace. There's a comfortably hard feeling to the pace that requires practice.

For competitive runners, AT pace is about 25 to 30 seconds per mile slower than 5K race pace (about 15 seconds per mile slower than 10K race pace) and corresponds to about 85 to 90 percent of maximum heart rate.

Workout #5: AT Run

Objective: To increase the athlete's acidosis threshold.

Description: On a measured and preferably flat cross country course or grass field, athletes run 3 to 6 miles (20 to 40 minutes) at AT pace. This is the most basic of AT workouts, but it is very effective for raising the athlete's acidosis threshold.

Coaching Points:
- It's important to keep the AT pace as steady as possible during these workouts, with little to no fluctuation in pace. The point is to raise the athlete's blood lactate level to it's threshold value (which indicates the onset of acidosis), and then hold it there for the duration of the workout.
- Since it's tempting for athletes to push the pace during these AT workouts, emphasize the purpose of the workout and the importance to remain aerobic.
- To practice the final push to the finish line during races, athletes may pick up the pace (albeit slightly) during the last quarter-mile of the AT run.

Workout #6: Long AT Run

Objective: To increase the acidosis threshold while running farther to prepare for longer races.

Description: Sometimes, it's beneficial to run a bit slower than AT pace to accommodate a longer distance, which comes with it the psychological demand of holding a comfortably hard pace for an extended time. Athletes run 6 to 10 miles (40 to 60 minutes) at 10 to 20 seconds per mile slower than AT pace.

Coaching Point: Athletes should view this workout as a way to increase the length of their runs at near AT pace. Therefore, they should be close to their AT pace for the entire run.

Workout #7: Handicap AT Run

Objective: To increase acidosis-threshold pace during a fun workout in which everyone finishes at the same time.

Description: Athletes run 3 miles at AT pace, with the slowest runner starting first and the fastest runner starting last. After the first runner begins, each subsequent runner begins after the amount of time has elapsed that equals the difference in AT paces over the entire run. For example, if Runners A, B, and C have AT paces of 5:30, 5:45, and 6:10, respectively, Runner C starts first, followed 1 minute and 15 seconds later (25 seconds times 3 miles) by Runner B, and 2 minutes later (40 seconds times 3 miles) by Runner A. If all runners run at their correct AT paces, everyone should cross the finish line together. This workout puts both the faster and slower runners in a unique position—the faster runners get the opportunity to catch the slower runners, and the slower runners get the opportunity to know what it's like to lead and be chased. This workout can be made longer by calculating the correct handicapped time for each runner.

Coaching Point: Don't let the faster runners "chase" the slower runners by running faster than their correct AT paces.

Workout #8: AT Serial Runs

Objective: To make the AT run both physically and psychologically easier while still obtaining the same benefit of continuous running at AT pace.

Description: This workout breaks the continuous AT run into shorter runs with recovery periods. Athletes run 2 to 4 x 10 to 15 minutes (about 2 miles) at AT pace with 3 to 5 minutes rest.

Coaching Point: If athletes have heart rate monitors, AT runs should be run at 85 to 90 percent of maximum heart rate.

Workout #9: AT Intervals

Objective: To make the AT workout both physically and psychologically easier and to increase the distance athletes can run at AT pace, you can design the workout in an interval format.

Description: Athletes run 3 to 6 x 1 mile at AT pace with a one-minute rest or 6 to 8 x 1,000 meters at AT pace with a one-minute rest.

Coaching Points:
- While it is tempting for athletes to run faster when the work periods are shorter, the purpose of this workout is the same as it is with continuous AT runs—to increase the acidosis threshold. Therefore, make sure athletes do not run any faster when doing AT intervals as when they do AT runs. They should still run at AT pace.
- Each repetition should be run at exactly the same pace, completing all reps within 1 to 2 seconds of each other, assuming you're using the same part of the cross country course for each rep.
- AT intervals are "rhythm" workouts. Encourage athletes to try to find the rhythm within each repetition.
- Athletes should focus on having their feet land directly beneath their center of gravity and "roll" through each step to maintain a solid rhythm.

Workout #10: AT+ Intervals

Objective: To add slightly more stress to the AT intervals as a way to further stimulate changes in AT pace to reach a faster speed.

Description: This version of AT intervals is run slightly faster than AT pace (hence the plus). Athletes run 2 sets of 4 x 1,000 meters (or 800 meters for less talented runners) at 5 to 10 seconds per mile faster than AT pace with 45 seconds rest and 2 minutes rest between sets.

Coaching Point: Make sure athletes don't get carried away with this workout. The pace must be only slightly faster than AT pace. If AT runs and AT intervals feel "comfortably hard," AT+ intervals should feel "hard but comfortable."

Workout #11: AT/LSD Combo Run

Objective: To increase the acidosis threshold while learning to combat fatigue in long cross country races.

Description: A twist on the 1970s term, "long slow distance," athletes run medium-long runs with a portion run at AT pace: 10 to 12 miles easy + 2 to 4 miles at AT pace. You can also mix the AT-paced running throughout the workout, such as 3 miles easy + 3 miles at AT pace + 5 miles easy + 3 miles at AT pace.

Coaching Points:
- These workouts are demanding, so it is necessary that athletes run the easy portions easy.
- When running the AT portion at the end of the run, the athletes' heart rates may exceed their normal AT heart rates (85 to 90 percent maximum heart rate) due to the cardiac drift associated with longer runs, especially on hot and humid days. However, athletes should not slow down their AT pace in an attempt to bring the higher heart rate down. Rather, they should focus on maintaining their correct AT paces.

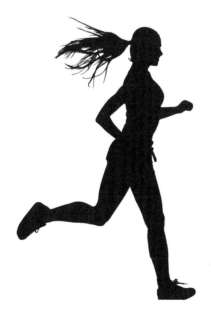

4

$\dot{V}O_2$max Training

You can't be a runner or distance running coach without hearing about $\dot{V}O_2$max. But what really is $\dot{V}O_2$max? Although it sounds like a disease ("Honey, you better stay away. I have $\dot{V}O_2$max."), $\dot{V}O_2$max is the maximum volume of oxygen that your muscles can consume per minute. It is therefore referred to as *aerobic power* since it's a measure of the *rate* at which oxygen is consumed.

$\dot{V}O_2$max is considered to be the best single indicator of a person's aerobic fitness. Although a high $\dot{V}O_2$max alone is not enough to attain elite-level performances, it gains athletes access into the club. An athlete simply cannot attain a high level of performance without a high $\dot{V}O_2$max. Owing to the importance of this physiological determinant of performance, $\dot{V}O_2$max is the most often measured variable in exercise physiology.

While $\dot{V}O_2$max can initially be improved by increasing the athlete's weekly running mileage, it is best improved with interval workouts, with the work periods lasting 3 to 5 minutes. During the work periods, athletes should run at or very close to $\dot{V}O_2$max (Figure 4-1). Repeatedly reaching and sustaining $\dot{V}O_2$max during the work periods represents the stimulus for its improvement. If the recovery period is short (equal to or less than the time spent running), oxygen consumption ($\dot{V}O_2$) will not decrease all the way back down to its resting value. This is a good thing, because the next work period will then begin with the $\dot{V}O_2$ elevated. $\dot{V}O_2$ will then rise again during the subsequent work period, to a point higher than during the first work period. If planned right, $\dot{V}O_2$ will reach $\dot{V}O_2$max after a couple of work periods, which is the goal of the workout. These workouts are difficult, as not only is oxygen being consumed at its fastest rate, but there is also a considerable oxygen-independent (anaerobic) contribution to the workout.

For competitive runners, $\dot{V}O_2$max pace is approximately 3,000-meter or two-mile race pace or 10 to 15 seconds per mile faster than 5K race pace, and corresponds to about 95 to 100 percent of maximum heart rate.

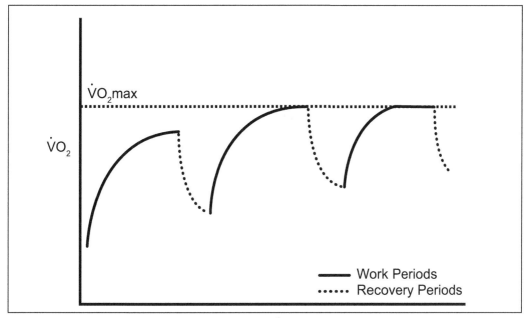

Figure 4-1. The increase in oxygen consumption ($\dot{V}O_2$) during an interval workout. The goal is to reach and sustain $\dot{V}O_2$max during each work period. In this example, $\dot{V}O_2$max is reached briefly during the second work period and is reached sooner during the third work period due to the elevated $\dot{V}O_2$ at the beginning of the third work period.

Workout #12: 800-Meter Repeats

Objective: To increase $\dot{V}O_2$max.

Description: On a cross country course or grass field, measure 800 meters. Athletes run 5 to 6 x 800 meters at their $\dot{V}O_2$max pace, with a 1:≤1 work-to-rest ratio. For example, a runner who can run two miles in 12:00 (6:00 pace) should run each 800-meter repeat in 3:00 with 2:30 to 3:00 jog recovery.

Coaching Point: It's important that the recovery periods remain active with light jogging to keep oxygen consumption ($\dot{V}O_2$) elevated throughout the workout. Doing so helps the athletes to reach $\dot{V}O_2$max earlier in the next work period, so that more time can be spent running at $\dot{V}O_2$max.

Workout #13: 1,000-Meter Repeats

Objective: To increase $\dot{V}O_2$max in runners whose $\dot{V}O_2$max pace is faster than 6:00 pace.

Description: Athletes run 5 to 6 x 1,000 meters at their $\dot{V}O_2$max pace, with a 1:≤1 work-to-rest ratio. For example, a runner who can run two miles in 11:00 (5:30 pace) should run each 1,000-meter repeat in 3:26 with 3:00 to 3:25 jog recovery.

Coaching Point: Athletes can monitor $\dot{V}O_2$max intervals with heart rate, reaching 95 to 100 percent of maximum heart rate over at least the last minute of each work period.

Workout #14: 1,200-Meter Repeats

Objective: To further increase $\dot{V}O_2$max by increasing the length of the work periods.

Description: Athletes run 4 to 5 x 1,200 meters at their $\dot{V}O_2$max pace, with a 1:≤1 work-to-rest ratio. For example, a runner who can run two miles in 11:00 (5:30 pace) should run each 1,200-meter repeat in 4.07 with 3:30 to 4.00 jog recovery.

Coaching Point: In an effort to equate the stress of workouts between runners of different abilities, use this hierarchy of strategies:
- Decrease the length of each work period for slower runners (or increase the length of each work period for faster runners) to make the duration of each work period the same between runners.
- Decrease the number of repetitions for slower runners (or increase the number of repetitions for faster runners) to make the total time spent running at $\dot{V}O_2$max pace the same.
- Increase the duration of the recovery period for slower runners (or decrease the duration of the recovery period for faster runners) to make the work-to-rest ratio the same.

Workout #15: Mile Repeats

Objective: To increase $\dot{V}O_2$max while running farther to prepare for longer races.

Description: Sometimes, it's beneficial to run a bit slower than $\dot{V}O_2$max pace to accommodate a longer distance, which comes with it the psychological demand of holding a hard pace for an extended time. For athletes training for longer races, the slight tradeoff of running a bit slower to extend the distance is often worth it. Athletes run 3 to 4 x 1 mile at 95 percent of their $\dot{V}O_2$max pace, with a 1:≤1 work-to-rest ratio. For example, a runner who can run two miles in 10:30 (5:15 pace) should run each mile repeat in 5:30 with 3:30 to 4:00 jog recovery. To calculate 95 percent $\dot{V}O_2$max pace, convert the athlete's $\dot{V}O_2$max pace into minutes, then multiply by 0.05, add that result to the original time, and then convert back into minutes and seconds. For the above runner: (5.25 minutes x 0.05) + 5.25 minutes = 5.5 minutes = 5:30 pace.

Coaching Point: This workout is tough and is best done in groups in which athletes can take turns leading each repetition.

Workout #16: 200-Meter Repeats

Objective: To increase $\dot{V}O_2$max using shorter intervals, which allows athletes to complete a greater total distance at $\dot{V}O_2$max pace.

Description: Athletes run 30 to 40 x 200 meters at their $\dot{V}O_2$max pace, with a 1:≤1 work-to-rest ratio. For example, a runner who can run two miles in 11:00 (5:30 pace) should run each 200-meter repeat in 41 seconds with 20 seconds jog recovery.

Coaching Points:
- Short intervals (< 2 minutes) can also improve $\dot{V}O_2$max, as long as you keep the recovery periods very short and active to keep oxygen consumption ($\dot{V}O_2$) elevated throughout the workout.
- Although it is tempting to run faster when the work periods are shorter, the pace should be the same regardless of their length (e.g., 200 meters vs. 1,000 meters) when the goal of the workout is to train $\dot{V}O_2$max.

Workout #17: 400-Meter Repeats

Objective: To increase $\dot{V}O_2$max using shorter intervals in runners whose $\dot{V}O_2$max pace is faster than 6:00 pace.

Description: Athletes run 15 to 20 x 400 meters at their $\dot{V}O_2$max pace, with a 1:≤1 work-to-rest ratio. For example, a runner who can run two miles in 11:00 (5:30 pace) should run each 400-meter repeat in 82 seconds with 40 seconds jog recovery.

Coaching Point: Many athletes run the first couple of repetitions too fast, making subsequent repetitions slower and slower. Make sure athletes run the correct pace from the beginning of the workout so that each rep can be run in the exact same time.

Workout #18: $\dot{V}O_2$max Ladder

Objective: To increase $\dot{V}O_2$max while running different distances and adding variety to the workout.

Description: Athletes run two sets of 800, 1,000, and 1,200 meters at their $\dot{V}O_2$max pace, with a 1:≤1 work-to-rest ratio. For example, a runner who can run two miles in 10:00 (5:00 pace) should run 2:30, 3:07, and 3:45 for the 800, 1,000, and 1,200 meters, respectively, with 2:30 to 3:00 jog recovery. For college women who race 6K, this workout will cover the entire course.

Coaching Point: Athletes should aim to run the work periods of the second set in the exact same time as the work periods of the first set.

Workout #19: $\dot{V}O_2$max Cut-Downs

Objective: To increase $\dot{V}O_2$max while running a greater range of distances and incorporating different percentages of $\dot{V}O_2$max in the same workout.

Description: Athletes run one to two sets of 1,600, 1,200, 1,000, 800, and 400 meters at 5K race pace for the 1,600, $\dot{V}O_2$max pace for the 1,200, 1,000, and 800, and faster than $\dot{V}O_2$max pace for the 400, with a 1:≤1 work-to-rest ratio. For example, a runner who can run 5K in 18:30 (5:58 pace) should run 1,600 meters in 5:58, 1,200 meters in 4:17 to 4:21 (5:43 to 5:48 pace), 1,000 meters in 3:34 to 3:37 (5:43 to 5:48 pace), 800 meters in 2:52 to 2:54 (5:43 to 5:48 pace), and 400 meters in 84 seconds (5:38 pace), with 3:00 to 3:30 jog recovery.

Coaching Point: Since this workout gets easier with each repetition, don't let the athletes get carried away by running too fast, especially with the 400 meters at the end.

Workout #20: $\dot{V}O_2$max Pyramid

Objective: To increase $\dot{V}O_2$max while running different distances and adding variety to the workout.

Description: Athletes run 800, 1,000, 1,200, 1,000, and 800 meters at their $\dot{V}O_2$max pace, with a 1:≤1 work-to-rest ratio. For example, a runner who can run two miles in 10:45 (5:22 pace) should run 2:41, 3:21, and 4:01 for the 800, 1,000, and 1,200 meters, respectively, with 2:30 to 3:30 jog recovery. For high school boys and girls who race 5K, this workout will cover nearly the entire course.

Coaching Point: The combination of different distances and different paces for each athlete can cause mayhem on the cross country course. Therefore, to have an organized workout in which each athlete achieves the objective, make sure each athlete knows what pace he is supposed to run for each distance.

Workout #21: Handicap $\dot{V}O_2$max Intervals

Objective: To increase $\dot{V}O_2$max by adding variety and fun to the workout and giving faster and slower runners something to motivate them.

Description: Athletes run 800 to 1,200 meters at $\dot{V}O_2$max pace, with the slowest runner starting first and the fastest runner starting last. After the first runner begins, each subsequent runner begins after the amount of time has elapsed that equals the difference in $\dot{V}O_2$max paces over the distance of the work period. For example, if running 1,000-meter repeats, and Runners A, B, and C have $\dot{V}O_2$max paces of 5:30, 5:45, and 6:10 (equaling 3:26, 3:35, and 3:51 for 1,000 meters), respectively, Runner C starts first, followed 16 seconds later by Runner B, and 25 seconds later by Runner A. If all runners run their correct $\dot{V}O_2$max paces, everyone should complete each 1,000-meter repeat together.

Variation: The top one or two runners run just slightly faster than $\dot{V}O_2$max pace so they catch the slower runners before the end of the rep (about 50 to 100 meters before the finish). Each runner caught must try to keep up with the passing runner until the end of the rep. Be careful not to make the pace too much faster than $\dot{V}O_2$max pace for the top runners, otherwise the workout will be too difficult for the top runners and the slower runners will get caught too early and have a difficult time picking up the pace for the remainder of the rep.

Coaching Point: This workout puts both the faster and slower runners in a unique position—the faster runners get the opportunity to catch the slower runners, and the slower runners get the opportunity to know what it's like to lead and be chased. This workout can be altered for any work period distance by calculating the correct handicapped time for each runner.

Workout #22: AT Run/$\dot{V}O_2$max Intervals Mix

Objective: To increase acidosis threshold and $\dot{V}O_2$max by combining AT-paced running with $\dot{V}O_2$max-paced running and to practice running harder off of a comfortably hard pace.

Description: Athletes run 2 to 3 miles at AT pace + 3 to 4 x 800 to 1,000 meters at $\dot{V}O_2$max pace with a 1:1 work-to-rest ratio. For example, a runner who can run 5K in 18:00 should run 2 to 3 miles at 6:08 to 6:13 pace followed by 3:00 jog recovery + 3 to 4 x 1,000 meters in 3:28 to 3:31 (5:33 to 5:38 pace) with 3:30 jog recovery.

Coaching Point: This workout is set up by the AT-pace segment, so make sure athletes don't run the AT-pace segment too fast.

Workout #23: AT Intervals/$\dot{V}O_2$max Intervals Mix

Objective: To increase acidosis threshold and $\dot{V}O_2$max by combining AT-paced running with $\dot{V}O_2$max-paced running and to practice running harder off of a comfortably hard pace.

Description: For this workout, the AT segment is performed in an interval format rather than as a continuous run, making the workout slightly easier than Workout #22: AT Run/$\dot{V}O_2$max Intervals Mix. Athletes run 3 x 1 mile at AT pace with 1:00 rest + 3 to 4 x 800 to 1,000 meters at $\dot{V}O_2$max pace with a 1:1 work-to-rest ratio. For example, a runner who can run 5K in 16:00 should run 3 x 1 mile in 5:29 to 5:34 with 1:00 rest + 3 to 4 x 1,000 meters in 3:03 to 3:06 (4:54 to 4:59 pace) with 3:00 jog recovery.

Coaching Point: Like Workout #22: AT Run/$\dot{V}O_2$max Intervals Mix, this workout is set up by the AT-pace segment, so make sure athletes don't run the AT-pace segment too fast, which is easy to do given the rest periods within the AT-pace segment.

Workout #24: AT+ Intervals/$\dot{V}O_2$max Intervals Mix

Objective: To increase acidosis threshold and $\dot{V}O_2$max by combining AT+-paced running with $\dot{V}O_2$max-paced running and to practice running harder off of an already hard but comfortable pace.

Description: For this workout, the AT intervals are performed at the "+" intensity described in Chapter 3, making the workout slightly harder than Workout #23: AT Intervals/$\dot{V}O_2$max Intervals Mix. Athletes run 3 to 4 x 1,000 meters at 5 to 10 seconds per mile faster than AT pace with 1:00 rest + 3 to 4 x 800 to 1,000 meters at $\dot{V}O_2$max pace with a 1:1 work-to-rest ratio. For example, a runner who can run 5K in 17:00 should run 3 to 4 x 1,000 meters in 3:31 to 3:38 (5:39 to 5:49 pace, which is 5 to 10 seconds per mile faster than the runner's AT pace of 5:49 to 5:54) with 1:00 rest + 3 to 4 x 1,000 meters in 3:16 to 3:19 (5:14 to 5:19 pace) with 3:15 jog recovery.

Coaching Point: Running at LT+ pace and $\dot{V}O_2$max pace requires a lot of control. This workout should be performed as part of the athletes' progression, after they have completed Workouts #22 and #23 a few times.

Workout #25: Time Trial

Objective: To increase $\dot{V}O_2$max using a time trial, to determine the fitness level of the athletes in the beginning of the cross country season, to practice race strategy, and to build the athlete's confidence in a relaxed, non-pressure situation.

Description: Athletes run one half to two thirds of the racing distance as fast as they can, preferably on the same course that they will be racing.

Coaching Point: A time trial, especially in the beginning of the season, will help determine the athletes' paces for workouts. Given their intensity, time trials or races of 3K to 5K can be used as a substitute for a $\dot{V}O_2$max workout.

5

Anaerobic Capacity Training

In addition to the large aerobic contribution to cross country races, there is also a significant involvement of anaerobic metabolism, since the races are run at a speed faster than the acidosis threshold for most runners. When running faster than the heart and blood flow can provide oxygen to the muscles, some of the energy for muscle contraction is regenerated through anaerobic, or what I call "oxygen-independent," means. When this happens, a number of problems begin to arise inside runners' muscles. Primary among them is that the muscles lose their ability to contract effectively because of an increase in hydrogen ions, which causes the muscle pH to decrease, a condition called acidosis. Acidosis has a number of nasty side effects: it inhibits the enzyme that breaks down the energy molecule (ATP) inside muscles, which decreases muscle contractile force; it inhibits the release of calcium (the trigger for muscle contraction) from its storage site in muscles; and it inhibits the production of ATP from the metabolic pathway glycolysis by inhibiting glycolysis' most important enzyme.

In addition to hydrogen ion accumulation, other metabolites accumulate when running fast, including potassium ions and the two constituents of ATP—ADP and inorganic phosphate (P_i), each of which causes a specific problem inside muscles, from inhibition of specific enzymes involved in muscle contraction to interference with muscles' electrical charges, ultimately leading to a decrease in muscle force production and running speed.

Given the many fatigue-inducing factors associated with oxygen-independent metabolism, it's important for runners to develop their anaerobic capacity once they have developed themselves as aerobically as possible. The purposes of anaerobic capacity training are to cause a high degree of muscle acidosis so that athletes enhance their buffering capacity, to increase the number of enzymes that catalyze the chemical reactions in anaerobic glycolysis (the energy system that breaks down blood glucose and muscle and liver glycogen to resynthesize ATP) so that glycolysis can regenerate

ATP more quickly for muscle contraction, and to increase running speed by recruiting fast-twitch muscle fibers.

Workout #26: 400-Meter Repeats

Objective: To increase anaerobic capacity.

Description: Athletes run 6 to 8 x 400 meters at mile race pace with a 1:1 work-to-rest ratio. For example, a runner who can run one mile in 5:00 should run each 400-meter repeat in 75 seconds with 75 seconds jog recovery.

Coaching Point: While any segment of a cross country course can be used for this workout, having athletes run fast over the last 400 meters of the course will provide them with a "memory," which will help them pick up the pace when they get to that point in their races. Conversely, don't have athletes do this workout over the first 400 meters of the course to prevent them from starting races too fast.

Workout #27: 600-Meter Repeats

Objective: To increase anaerobic capacity by working at the upper end of the work period duration.

Description: Athletes run 4 to 5 x 600 meters at mile race pace with a 1:1 work-to-rest ratio. For example, a runner who can run one mile in 5:30 should run each 600-meter repeat in 2:03 with 2:00 jog recovery.

Coaching Point: This workout is demanding. Try to get athletes to think of this workout as 400-meter repeats, with a 200 tacked on at the end.

Workout #28: 300-Meter Repeats

Objective: To increase anaerobic capacity by increasing the intensity that causes a high degree of acidosis.

Description: Athletes run two sets of 4 x 300 meters at 800-meter race pace with a 1:2 work-to-rest ratio. For example, a runner who can run 800 meters in 2:20 should run each 300-meter repeat in 52 to 53 seconds with 1:45 jog recovery and 5 minutes recovery between sets.

Coaching Point: The pace for these workouts is based on what the athlete can do on a cross country course, which is considerably slower than on the track, so you'll need to make an adjustment in pace. Don't use the athlete's mile or 800-meter time from the track and expect him to run that pace on a cross country course for these workouts.

Workout #29: Anaerobic Capacity Ladder

Objective: To increase anaerobic capacity while adding variety to the workout.

Description: Athletes run two to four sets of 300, 400, and 600 meters at their mile race pace, with a 1:1.5 work-to-rest ratio. For example, a runner who can run one mile in 5:30 should run 61 seconds, 82 seconds, and 2:03 for the 300, 400, and 600 meters, respectively, with 1:30 to 3:00 jog recovery (with the upper end of the recovery range following longer work periods) and 3:00 to 5:00 recovery between sets.

Coaching Point: Since this workout gets progressively harder within each set, make sure athletes don't run too fast for the 300 and 400. The pace should be the same for each repetition.

Workout #30: Anaerobic Capacity Pyramid

Objective: To increase anaerobic capacity while adding variety to the workout.

Description: Athletes run one to two sets of 300, 400, 600, 800, 600, 400, and 300 meters at their mile race pace, with a 1:1.5 work-to-rest ratio. For example, a runner who can run one mile in 5:10 should run 58 seconds, 77 seconds, 1:56, and 2:35 for the 300, 400, 600, and 800 meters, respectively, with 1:30 to 3:45 jog recovery (with the upper end of the recovery range following longer work periods) and 5:00 recovery between sets.

Coaching Point: In an effort to equate the stress of workouts between runners of different abilities, use this hierarchy of strategies:
- Decrease the length of each work period for slower runners (or increase the length of each work period for faster runners) to make the duration of each work period the same between runners.
- Decrease the number of repetitions for slower runners (or increase the number of repetitions for faster runners) to make the total time spent running at anaerobic capacity pace the same.
- Increase the duration of the recovery period for slower runners (or decrease the duration of the recovery period for faster runners) to make the work-to-rest ratio the same.

Workout #31: $\dot{V}O_2$max/Anaerobic Capacity Mix

Objective: To combine $\dot{V}O_2$max-paced running with anaerobic capacity work, to practice running fast off of already hard running, and to help develop a kick.

Description: Athletes run 3 to 4 x 800 to 1,000 meters at $\dot{V}O_2$max pace + 4 to 6 x 400 meters at mile race pace with a 1:1 work-to-rest ratio during the $\dot{V}O_2$max portion of the workout and a 1:2 work-to-rest ratio during the anaerobic capacity portion of the workout. For example, a runner who can run 5K in 17:00 should run 3 to 4 x 1,000 meters in 3:16 to 3:19 (5:14 to 5:19 pace) with 3:15 jog recovery + 4 to 6 x 400 meters in 73 to 74 seconds (4:54 pace) with 2:25 jog recovery.

Coaching Point: This workout is set up by the $\dot{V}O_2$max-pace segment, so make sure athletes don't run the $\dot{V}O_2$max-pace segment too fast.

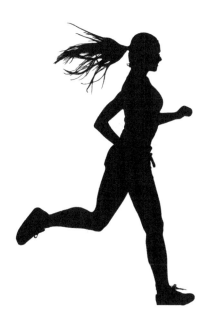

6

Hill Training

Hills are a big part of cross country running. Many cross country courses have hills that athletes must learn to navigate. Many races are won or lost on a hill.

Hill training has a number of advantages: it increases leg muscle power, it can be used as a great transition into more formal speedwork, it can improve the performance of the heart since heart rate can easily climb up to its maximum when running up a hill, and it uses the muscles of the legs, arms, and trunk in ways that are different from flat running.

Even though running uphill seems harder, it's the downhills that cause the biggest problems. The reason downhills are so tough is because of all the gravity-induced eccentric muscle contractions, during which muscle fibers are forced to lengthen, causing them to tear. The forces of impact and braking are also greater during downhill running and less during uphill running compared to running on a flat surface. Therefore, running downhill carries a greater risk of overuse injury compared to uphill or flat running. The good news is that damaging muscle fibers with eccentric contractions makes them heal back stronger, protecting them from future damage. While athletes can expect their muscles to be sore after the first time running downhill, subsequent downhill workouts will cause less soreness since running downhill has a prophylactic effect on muscle damage and soreness.

Since hill running uncouples the effort from the speed (i.e., athletes are running relatively slow even though they're working hard), the exact pace is not as important as the effort. Therefore, athletes should aim for a specific effort rather than a specific speed. Monitoring heart rate with a heart-rate monitor is a great way to make sure the athlete is working hard enough.

Workout #32: Hill Run

Objective: To get athletes used to running on hilly terrain in a continuous run.

Description: This workout is a basic trail/grass run of 4 to 8 miles that includes hills of varying lengths and grades. It should be used over the summer to prepare the athletes for more formal hill training during cross country season.

Coaching Point: Since the pace will fluctuate substantially during the run, athletes should focus on maintaining an even effort rather than pace.

Workout #33: Long Hill Repeats

Objective: To increase cardiovascular fitness and leg muscle power.

Description: Athletes run 5 to 6 x half-mile uphill at 5K race pace effort with a jog back down as recovery. The slope of the hill should be 5 to 8 percent.

Coaching Point: This workout can take the place of one of the $\dot{V}O_2$max workouts in Chapter 4. Hills that take at least 3 minutes to climb can be used to increase $\dot{V}O_2$max since the athlete's heart rate and stroke volume (the volume of blood pumped by the heart per beat) can rise up to their maximum values when running hard up a hill. (In a laboratory setting, the $\dot{V}O_2$max test is almost always performed using an increase in treadmill grade as a way to use more muscle mass and get athletes to reach their $\dot{V}O_2$max.)

Workout #34: Short Hill Repeats

Objective: To develop anaerobic capacity and muscle power of the quadriceps, gluteus maximus, hip flexors, and calves.

Description: Athletes sprint 8 to 10 x 100 meters uphill with jog back down as recovery. For this workout, the slope should be steep (15 to 20 percent).

Coaching Point: When running uphill, athletes should exaggerate their arm swing, lean into the hill, and focus on pushing off with the ball of the foot.

Workout #35: Uphill/Downhill Repeats

Objective: To mix uphill and downhill running, which is great practice for cross country racing since many courses have both uphills and downhills.

Description: Athletes run 4 x half-mile uphill + quarter-mile downhill (2 to 3 percent slope) at 5K race pace effort with 3 minutes jog recovery.

Coaching Points:
- Add downhills to the training a little at a time. Start with a short, gradual slope of about 2 to 3 percent, and progress to steeper and longer descents.
- Since athletes are running faster on downhills compared to the flat or uphill sections of cross country courses, they have less time to decide on foot placement, so tell athletes to look ahead a few steps so they can prepare since the footing on cross country courses is often unreliable.

Workout #36: Short Downhill Repeats

Objective: To increase speed and get athletes used to the eccentric contractions associated with downhill running, which will protect them from muscle-fiber damage when running downhill in a race.

Description: Athletes run 8 to 10 x 100 meters nearly all-out on a 2 to 3 percent downhill slope with jog back uphill as recovery.

Coaching Points:
- When running downhill, athletes should shorten their strides to prevent overstriding and emphasize a quicker leg turnover, which will keep momentum going forward. They should feel like it's controlled falling.
- Given the stressful nature of downhill running, treat downhill workouts as hard sessions and give athletes time to recover with two to three days of easy running afterward. Be sure to back off of the hills in the final couple weeks before a race.
- Given the fast speeds attained in this workout (and thus a diminished time to spot foot placement), use a smooth stretch of grass for short downhill repeats so athletes don't trip or roll their ankles.

Workout #37: Hill Accelerators

Objective: To help athletes learn how to run hills aggressively and defeat their competitors, as they will be accelerating when their opponents are laboring at the top of the hill.

Description: Athletes run 4 to 8 x 200- to 400-meter hill, running the bottom of the hill at race-pace effort (leading into the hill from a 200-meter flat section at race pace) and accelerating the last 50 meters of the hill and 100 meters from the top, with jog back down as recovery.

Coaching Points:
- Athletes should aim for the same time for all reps.
- The focus of this workout is the acceleration at the top of the hill, which is opposite to the recovery that athletes naturally want to take at the top of a hill.
- When athletes get to the top of the hill, remind them to pump their arms to help them accelerate and lengthen their strides, which will have shortened on the hill.

Workout #38: Hill Bounding

Objective: To increase leg muscle power.

Description: Using an exaggerated running motion, athletes bound six to eight times up a steep hill (15 to 20 percent slope) for 40 to 50 meters and jog back down.

Coaching Point: Athletes should try to achieve as much horizontal distance with each bound. Athletes should focus on fully extending the push-off leg and driving the knee of the forward leg up.

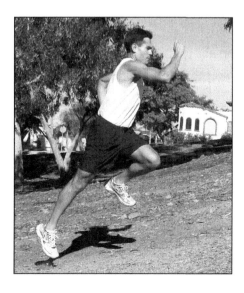

7

Fartlek Training

Fartlek, from the Swedish words *fart* (meaning "speed") and *lek* (meaning "play"), dates back to 1937, when it was developed by Swedish coach Gösta Holmér. It was used as part of Sweden's military training. Fartleks are continuous runs during which athletes pick up the pace at different times, when they reach specific landmarks, or just based on how they feel. Distances, speeds, and recovery periods may vary within the same workout. Fartleks can be used to learn different paces, work on team tactics, respond to other runners' surges, add variety and fun to athletes' training, and as a transition into more formal speedwork.

Workout #39: The Classic Fartlek

Objective: To play with changes in speed and have fun while doing a quality workout determined by effort.

Description: Depending on ability and level of training, athletes run 3 to 8 miles through park trails and grass fields, changing the pace throughout the run based on how they feel. For this workout, there is no set paces or times, and athletes shouldn't even wear watches other than to keep track of the total time they're running.

Coaching Point: For young, less-experienced runners, this workout is a low-pressure, non-intimidating way to introduce faster-paced running. Runners shouldn't focus on pace. Just have them listen to their bodies and run accordingly.

Workout #40: The Classic Aerobic Fartlek

Objective: To play with changes in speed up to the acidosis threshold.

Description: A variation of the classic fartlek, athletes run 3 to 8 miles, picking up the pace according to how they feel, with all of the speeds used throughout the run being aerobic, with the acidosis threshold being the fastest speed.

Coaching Point: Emphasize the importance of this workout remaining aerobic so athletes don't push the pace. The use of a heart-rate monitor during this workout is beneficial to prevent running too fast. Have athletes set the heart-rate monitor to beep at their acidosis-threshold heart rates (about 85 percent of maximum heart rate).

Workout #41: The Classic Anaerobic Fartlek

Objective: To play with changes in speed above the acidosis threshold.

Description: Another variation of the classic fartlek, athletes run 3 to 8 miles, picking up the pace according to how they feel, with all of the pick-ups used throughout the run being anaerobic, all being faster than acidosis-threshold pace, with only the recovery periods between pick-ups being aerobic.

Coaching Point: This workout can be used as a transition into more formal anaerobic work. As with the other classic fartleks, the pick-ups and recovery periods are self-selected by the athletes based on their fitness levels and how they feel.

Workout #42: The 3-2-1 Fartlek

Objective: To add structure to the classic fartlek and learn how to pick up the pace at designated times rather than by feel.

Description: Athletes run 3 to 6 miles, picking up the pace for 3 minutes, 2 minutes, and 1 minute with equal time jog recovery, and repeat this 3-2-1 pattern throughout the run.

Coaching Point: Have athletes do this workout in a group, with teammates taking turns leading the pick-ups.

Workout #43: The Ladder Fartlek

Objective: To add structure to the classic fartlek and play with different lengths of hard efforts.

Description: After an adequate warm-up, athletes run 1 minute, 2 minutes, 3 minutes, 4 minutes, and 5 minutes hard with equal time jog recovery. More advanced runners can do two sets.

Variation: For a sprint ladder fartlek, athletes do three to four sets of 30-second sprints, 1 minute sprint, 1:30 sprint, and 2 minutes sprint with 2 minutes jog recovery.

Coaching Point: Since this workout gets progressively difficult, remind athletes to not start out too fast.

Workout #44: The Pyramid Fartlek

Objective: To add structure to the classic fartlek, getting progressively difficult and then progressively less difficult.

Description: After an adequate warm-up, athletes run 1 minute, 2 minutes, 3 minutes, 4 minutes, 3 minutes, 2 minutes, and 1 minute hard with equal time jog recovery.

Variation: Athletes run 2 minutes, 4 minutes, 5 minutes, 4 minutes, and 2 minutes hard with 3 minutes jog recovery.

Coaching Point: Pair up runners based on ability and encourage them to help one another throughout the run.

Workout #45: Tee to Green

Objective: To structure the classic fartlek based on landmarks.

Description: On a golf course, starting at the first tee, athletes run hard from the tee to the green, with a jog recovery from the green to the next tee. Athletes run as many holes of the golf course as is reasonable for their ability and fitness level.

Coaching Point: Given the distance between a golf course green and the next tee compared to between a tee and its green, the recovery periods are short in this workout compared to the pick-ups, so remind athletes to be careful about pushing the pace early in the workout and run very easy during the short recovery periods.

8

Strategy and Tactics Training

Cross country racing presents unique strategic opportunities because athletes can take advantage of the natural terrain of cross country courses. For example, athletes who have a lot of strength can use the hills to their advantage by surging up the hills. Also, when making turns on a cross country course, trailing runners often cannot see a runner after he has made the turn because of trees or bushes. These blind turns, what I call "hot spots," are a great place for making a short surge immediately after making the turn. Then, when the trailing runner makes the same turn, he is surprised and, more importantly, psychologically defeated, to see the runner farther ahead.

While the best way to run a race to achieve the fastest possible time is to maintain an even pace the whole race and even run the second half slightly faster than the first (called "negative splits"), sometimes the course topography and terrain and race strategy dictate that athletes change the pace during the race to challenge their competitors. Starts, negative splits, a fast first mile, quick changes in pace, accelerating up or down a hill, blocking runners on narrow paths, multiple mid-race surges, an early kick, and pack running are all strategies used by athletes and teams to separate themselves from the competition and win races. Therefore, it's important to practice these strategies in training so that athletes can execute them in races and can respond when employed by their competitors.

Workout #46: Practice Starts

Objective: To practice race starts.

Description: The start is an important part of a cross country race, especially at big meets where a few hundred runners can be on the start line. With all the chaos, adrenaline, and excitement that surrounds the start of a cross country race, it's very easy for runners to go out too fast, lose their teammates in the scramble, and be taken out of their race plan. Set up an area that resembles the first 400 meters of the course your athletes will race. You can also use your home course. Set the runners on the start line in the configuration they will use in the race. Choose one runner to lead the group out, with the others following his lead. Give each runner another teammate to follow. Athletes run 5 to 10 practice starts (400 meters), with each runner focusing on the job to follow the designated leader, making sure to stay within touching distance of that teammate. This simple workout provides an order and calmness to what can otherwise be total chaos.

Coaching Point: Make sure your athletes duplicate this workout in their race so they know exactly what to do at the start and who they will be near.

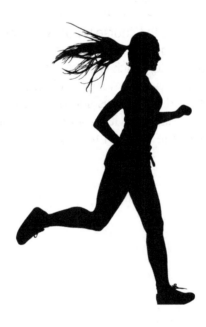

Workout #47: The Negative Split

Objective: To practice running the second half of a workout faster than the first to prepare for races.

Description: To achieve the best possible racing time, the second half of a race should be equal to or slightly faster than the first half (called "negative splits"). To negative split a race, athletes need an accurate knowledge of their fitness level, confidence to stick to their plan when others have taken the early pace out too fast, a good dose of self-restraint, and the ability to control their emotions at the start. Sometimes, negative splitting is not possible in cross country races given the nature and terrain of the course. However, if the course is flat or has a repeating loop, negative splitting is possible. To practice running negative splits, athletes run 1 mile at acidosis-threshold pace, followed by half the remaining race distance at race pace (typically 5K for high school boys and girls, 6K for college women, and 8K to 10K for college men). For example, high school runners should run 1 mile at acidosis-threshold pace + 1 mile at 5K-race pace. College men should run 1 mile at acidosis-threshold pace + 2 miles at 8K-race pace.

Variation: Athletes run 3 to 4 x 1 mile with 3 minutes jog recovery between each mile, running the first mile at acidosis-threshold pace, the second mile 10 seconds per mile faster than acidosis-threshold pace, the third mile at race pace, and the fourth mile 10 seconds per mile faster than race pace.

Coaching Point: Runners will race the way they practice. If they always run too fast in the beginning of their workouts, they will do the same thing in their races. Remind athletes that the goal of the workout is to run the second half faster than the first, so they need to run with their heads the first half and control themselves.

Workout #48: Fast First Mile

Objective: To learn how to race off a fast early pace.

Description: Oftentimes, good runners will take the early pace out fast to set themselves apart from their competitors, take the kick out of their competitors' legs, and break the race open early. For this workout, athletes run 1 mile 10 to 15 seconds per mile faster than race pace (5K for high school boys and girls, 6K for college women, and 8K to 10K for college men), followed by 2 to 3 miles at acidosis-threshold pace.

Variation: Athletes run 1 mile 10 to 15 seconds per mile faster than race pace + 1 mile at race pace + 1 to 2 miles at acidosis-threshold pace.

Coaching Point: This workout is tough, so athletes need to be ready for it. Try to do the workout over the course they will be racing.

Workout #49: Hill Accelerations

Objective: To practice running hills fast, and to use hills to break open races.

Description: Athletes run 3 to 6 miles on a hilly course, accelerating up each hill and maintaining a comfortable pace on the flat and downhill portions.

Coaching Point: When accelerating up the hills, athletes should focus on pumping their arms and continue to accelerate until they have run over the crest of the hill.

Workout #50: The Surge Run

Objective: To practice reacting to other runners' surges.

Description: Break your team into groups with runners of similar abilities. Each group runs together for 4 to 5 miles, with one runner being designated as the pacesetter whose job it is to surge at different points in the run. When the pacesetter surges, the other runners practice reacting to the surge and picking up the pace to match the pacesetter.

Variation: Instead of having just one pacesetter, each runner in the group can surge at any time, with the other runners reacting to the surge and covering the move.

Coaching Point: To be effective, surges should start abruptly and end gradually, with surges lasting at least 20 to 30 seconds.

Workout #51: Surging Intervals

Objective: To practice surging and return to race pace following the surge.

Description: Athletes run 5 x 600 meters on a 200-meter loop, running race pace for the first loop, 5 to 10 seconds per mile faster than race pace for the second loop, and returning to race pace for the third loop, with a 200-meter loop jog recovery. For example, a runner who can run 5K in 19:00 (6:07 pace) would run the first 200-meter loop in 45.9 seconds (6:07 pace), the second 200-meter loop in 44.8 to 45.4 seconds (5:58 to 6:03 pace), and the third 200-meter loop in 45.9 seconds (6:07 pace).

Coaching Point: Since it's difficult to return to race pace following a surge, remind athletes to stay focused throughout each repetition and not allow the pace to drop too much after surging.

Workout #52: The Early Kick

Objective: To practice kicking early for races.

Description: This workout can be done during an acidosis threshold or similar type of tempo run. The team runs their racing distance (5K to 10K) in a pack on the cross country course at AT pace or slightly faster (if the team includes many runners of varying abilities, they can be broken up into groups of similar abilities), with one runner being designated as the kicker (with only the coach and the kicker knowing who the kicker is). The kicker starts his kick at a pre-planned place on the course (far enough out from the finish to serve the purpose of an early kick). When the kicker kicks, it's his job to pull away from the pack and the job of each of the other runners to try to stay with the kicker. Throughout the season, each runner on the team should have a chance to be the kicker.

Variation: To more closely simulate kicking off of race pace, the athletes can run at race pace instead of AT pace, with the distance of the run shortened (for example, if the athletes race 5K, this workout can be done over a two-mile course).

Coaching Point: Make sure the kicker doesn't simply sprint away from everyone in the last 100 meters. This workout is about developing a kick that can begin as early as can be held, so it's better to run at 90 percent for 600 meters than 100 percent for 100 meters.

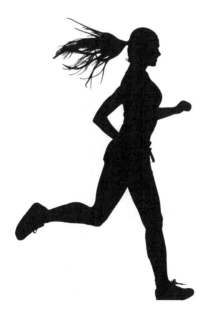

Workout #53: Race Divisions

Objective: To divide the race distance into equal parts to focus on each part of the course.

Description: This workout divides the race distance into more manageable parts, such as 800s for a 5K (high school boys and girls), 1,000s for a 6K (college women), or 1,000s or 1,600s for an 8K (college men). If the race distance is a 5K, athletes run 6 x 800 meters + 1 x 200 meters (= 5,000 meters) at slightly faster than race pace, jogging for equal time as recovery. The final 200 meters can be run fast to mimic the race situation. The number of repetitions in the workout should equal the race distance. Thus, college women who race 6K should run 6 x 1,000 meters and college men who race 8K should run either 8 x 1,000 meters or 5 x 1,600 meters. This is a similar workout to the $\dot{V}O_2$max intervals, however it's presented differently to the athletes as a way to prepare them for the racing distance. It's much easier for athletes to think they must run hard for six 800-meter repeats with no rest in between than to think they must run hard for 3.1 miles. Running six 800s faster than race pace with just a few minutes recovery between each will give them confidence for the race.

Coaching Point: The focus of this workout is the second half, just like it is in a race. Explain to the athletes that the first half of the workout is to get them fatigued going into the second half, and that they should focus on trying to make the second half reps as fast as those of the first half because it is during those second half reps (just like during the second half of the race) that they can do the most damage to their competitors.

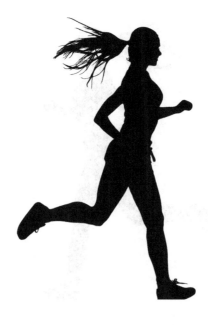

Workout #54: Pack Running

Objective: To practice running in a pack.

Description: The key to acquiring a low score and having a successful cross country team is to get all of the runners on your team to cross the finish line as close to one another (and to the front of the race) as possible. Therefore, you want as few runners from other teams to cross the finish line between your team's runners. During an acidosis-threshold (tempo) run, athletes run the first 2 to 3 miles together in a pack as fast as possible while keeping the whole varsity five- to seven-member team together. The faster runners should not run away from the slower runners, and the slower runners must do whatever they can to stay with the pack (or at least within arm's reach of the pack). If there is too much of a difference in performance level between the top five or seven runners on your team for them to run together in one group, divide the team into smaller groups so they can stay together. After running the first 2 to 3 miles together, the team can then fall into their individual AT paces for the rest of the tempo run.

Coaching Point: Remind athletes that, for this workout to have its intended effect, they have to really work together for the first 2 to 3 miles, which will be slightly faster than AT pace for the slower runners and slightly slower than AT pace for the faster runners.

Workout #55: Goal Race Pace Workout

Objective: To practice goal race pace.

Description: Athletes run 800-meter repeats at goal race pace (or a distance that allows them to run at goal race pace). Over time, the length of the work periods get longer as the athletes become more proficient at maintaining their goal race paces.

Coaching Point: While an athlete's race performances should be used to dictate the paces used in training, one drawback to this strategy is that the athlete never gets to experience what it feels like to run beyond his current fitness level. To circumvent this, athletes can mix in some goal race pace workouts into their training, although do not have it dominate the training strategy. Remember that the goal of training is to use the least stressful stimulus to cause the desired adaptation.

9

Cross Country Games

Games can be a great way to develop teamwork, make workouts fun, and teach athletes to race. Indeed, it was the English game, Hares and Hounds, that gave birth to the sport of cross country running. When using games to train cross country runners, it's important to remember the purpose of the workout and use a game that matches that purpose (or alter the game to meet the purpose) rather than use a game for the sheer sake of variety. Variety is good, since it keeps athletes motivated, but variety in the context of meeting the purpose of a workout so athletes can continue to improve is even better.

Workout #56: Hares and Hounds

Objective: To create a game out of a fartlek run.

Description: For a contemporary version of the English game that started the sport of cross country running, one or two runners are designated as the hares, with all of the other members of the team designated as the hounds. The hares run through woods, grass fields, and trails, hiding specific objects (flag, tennis ball, or any other small objects that can be held while running) and leaving a trail behind them (a bag of chalk or flour works well). Once the hares have enough of a head start, the hounds take off, following the trail left by the hares, searching for the hidden objects. The obvious goal of the game is for the hounds to find all of the hidden objects.

Coaching Point: To add an element of competition, the hounds can be divided into smaller teams of two or three runners who compete to find the hidden objects.

Workout #57: Blackjack Intervals

Objective: To create a game out of an interval workout using different paces.

Description: One athlete from the team picks a card from a deck of cards held by the coach. The length of the work period is determined by the chosen card. For example, if the athlete chooses a four from the deck of cards (regardless of the suit), the athletes run 400 meters. If the athlete chooses a 10, the athletes run 1,000 meters. During the subsequent recovery period, another card is chosen by another athlete to discover the length of the next work period. This pattern continues until 5 to 8 percent of the total weekly mileage is completed by the athletes. Work periods shorter than 700 meters are run at mile race pace, and periods 700 meters and longer are run at $\dot{V}O_2$max pace. Each recovery period is equal in time to the work period. A jack is equal to 1,200 meters, a queen is equal to 1,400 meters, and a king is equal to a mile (for distances longer than 1,200 meters, athletes may need to run a bit slower than $\dot{V}O_2$max pace to complete the workout). Aces and jokers can also be included, and if an ace is chosen, the athlete who chooses the card picks the distance the team will run. If a joker is chosen, the coach chooses the distance.

Coaching Point: This workout is fun for athletes, since they don't know what distances or how many repetitions they will run. Thus, it forces the athletes to focus solely on the next work period without thinking about the workout as a whole. Given the various distances covered, this workout requires that many distances be measured on the cross country course beforehand.

Workout #58: Blackjack Aerobic Intervals

Objective: To create a game out of a $\dot{V}O_2$max interval workout.

Description: One athlete from the team picks a card from a deck of cards held by the coach. The length of the work period is determined by the chosen card. For example, if the athlete chooses a 10 from the deck of cards (regardless of the suit), the athletes run 1,000 meters. During the subsequent recovery period, another card is chosen by another athlete to discover the length of the next work period. This pattern continues until 3 to 4 miles or 5 to 8 percent of the total weekly mileage is completed by the athletes. All work periods, regardless of their length, are run at $\dot{V}O_2$max pace and each recovery period is equal or slightly less than equal in time to the work period.

This is a fun way to do a $\dot{V}O_2$max interval workout, since the athletes don't know what distances or how many repetitions they will run. Thus, it forces the athletes to focus solely on the next work period without thinking about the workout as a whole. Given the various distances covered, this workout requires that many distances be measured on the cross country course beforehand.

Coaching Point: To keep the length of the work periods in agreement with the time range to target $\dot{V}O_2$max (3 to 5 minutes), stack the deck of cards in that favor by including only sevens or eights through kings. A jack is equal to 1,200 meters, a queen is equal to 1,400 meters, and a king is equal to a mile (if 1,400 meters or a mile exceeds the 5-minute upper limit, different distances can be chosen for the face cards). Aces and jokers can also be included, and if an ace is chosen, the athlete who chooses the card picks the distance the team will run. If a joker is chosen, the coach chooses the distance.

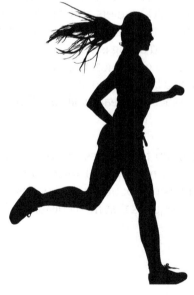

Workout #59: Blackjack Anaerobic Intervals

Objective: To create a game out of an anaerobic capacity interval workout.

Description: One athlete from the team picks a card from a deck of cards held by the coach. The length of the work period is determined by the chosen card. For example, if the athlete chooses a four from the deck of cards (regardless of the suit), the athletes run 400 meters. During the subsequent recovery period, another card is chosen by another athlete to discover the length of the next work period. This pattern continues until 2 miles or 5 to 8 percent of the total weekly mileage is completed by the athletes. All work periods, regardless of their length, are run at mile race pace and each recovery period is equal in time to the work period.

This workout is fun for athletes, since they don't know what distances or how many repetitions they will run. Thus, it forces the athletes to focus solely on the next work period without thinking about the workout as a whole. Given the various distances covered, this workout requires that many distances be measured on the cross country course beforehand.

Coaching Point: To keep the length of the work periods in agreement with the time range to target anaerobic capacity (45 seconds to about two minutes), stack the deck of cards in that favor by including only aces through sixes or sevens. If an ace is chosen, the athlete who chooses the card picks the distance the team will run. Jokers can also be included, with the coach choosing the distance if a joker is chosen.

Workout #60: Rabbit and Turtle

Objective: To create a game out of an Indian Run.

Description: A twist on the old-fashioned Indian Run, athletes run 3 to 5 miles in a straight line, with one runner behind the next. The runner at the end of the line sprints to the front. When the runner reaches the front, the next runner who is last in line sprints to the front. The entire line must stay together without large gaps forming between runners. If the pace of the entire line is deemed too slow by one of the runners, that runner can call out "Rabbit" to pick up the pace. If the pace is deemed too fast by one of the runners, that runner can call out "Turtle" to slow down the pace. The Indian Run continues in this manner, with the paces getting faster and slower with the commands of "Rabbit" and "Turtle," respectively.

Coaching Point: Remind athletes to work together to prevent large gaps from forming in the line. The number of pick-ups or slow-downs can be controlled by regulating the number of "Rabbits" and "Turtles" that can be used throughout the run.

Workout #61: Lions and Gazelles

*In Africa, every morning a gazelle awakens knowing that it
must outrun the fastest lion if it wants to stay alive.
Every morning a lion wakes up knowing that it must run
faster than the slowest gazelle, or it will starve to death.
It makes no difference whether you are a lion or a gazelle:
when the sun comes up, you had better be running.*
— African proverb

Objective: For faster runners to practice chasing and for slower runners to practice hanging with faster runners in the context of an acidosis-threshold workout.

Description: For this workout, the team is divided into groups based on ability, with the slower runners designated as the gazelles and the faster runners designated as the lions. The gazelles begin running at acidosis-threshold (tempo) pace, with the lions remaining behind. On the coach's signal, the lions are released and run at their acidosis-threshold pace until they catch the gazelles. When the lions catch the gazelles, the gazelles must surge to keep pace with passing lions for a predetermined amount of time. The gazelles then go back to running at acidosis-threshold pace until the next time a group of lions catches them.

Coaching Point: This workout stresses the importance of reacting to passing runners, practices the ability to "go with them" as they go by and, in so doing, increases the confidence of the slower runners that they can run with the faster runners.

Workout #62: Cross Country Relay

Objective: To create a relay out of an interval workout.

Description: The team is divided into compatible groups of three. Athletes run a predetermined distance for each relay leg (600 to 1,200 meters), handing off a baton to their team member. The recovery period is the time the other two members of the three-runner group are running their relay legs. The relay continues until each member of the group has run four or five relay legs. This workout is also called a *paarlauf*, which is German for "pair run."

Coaching Point: To make the workout more difficult, decrease the relay teams to two members, which will decrease the duration of the recovery periods.

Workout #63: Prediction Run

Objective: To practice running a specific time for a specific distance.

Description: With any type of workout (e.g., AT run or intervals), athletes try to predict their time, with the runner coming the closest to his predicted time winning something from the coach (e.g., a pizza dinner). Having the athletes predict what time they will run forces them to be more deliberate about the pace and to think about what they are doing.

Coaching Point: Remind athletes that the purpose is not to run as fast as they can, but rather to measure their effort over a given distance.

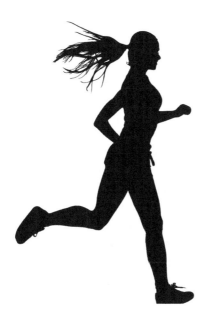

10

Supplemental Training

Supplemental training includes non-running activities, such as stretching, running form drills, circuit training, strength training, and plyometrics. While these activities may not have a direct impact on cross country running performance, they can improve the athlete's overall fitness, increase muscular strength, and reduce the chance of injury. Think of supplemental training as exercises and activities that prepare the runner for more formal training and the ability to handle greater training loads. In other words, supplemental training trains runners to train.

Stretching should be dynamic (rather than static) in nature, and focus on the important body parts for the cross country runner—hips (including glutes and hip flexors), quads, and hamstrings. While research does not fully support that stretching significantly reduces the risk of injuries or improves performance, stretching does improve flexibility and mobility, priming muscles to move dynamically through their full ranges of motion, which is important for cross country runners. The best stretching for cross country runners is dynamic (or active-isolated) stretching, during which the opposing muscle group is contracted, causing the stretched muscle group to relax so a greater stretch can be obtained as the limb is moved through its complete range of motion.

For young and inexperienced runners who are still developing their running skills, drills can help improve running mechanics and coordination. Running has an underrecognized neural component. Just as the repetition of the walking movements decreases the jerkiness of a toddler's walk to the point that it becomes smooth, the repetition of specific running movements can make a runner smoother and improves running economy, the amount of oxygen used to maintain a given speed. With countless repetitions, the athlete's motor unit (muscle fiber) recruitment pattern becomes ingrained, allowing for smoother running mechanics and a more efficient application of muscular force. In addition to the neural adaptation obtained with drills, drills can increase flexibility, since their dynamic action moves joints through an exaggerated range of motion.

Cross country runners can use circuit training for overall body conditioning early in the season. I prefer using body weight exercises rather than dumbbells since it's important for developing runners to increase their strength relative to their body weight so they can master the weight of their own bodies.

Any strength training that cross country runners do should be aimed at improving muscle strength without increasing muscle size (hypertrophy). Adding muscle mass reduces running economy (the amount of oxygen used to maintain a given pace) since it costs more oxygen to transport a heavier weight. (Young, physically immature runners may benefit from a slight increase in hypertrophy to make them stronger, more powerful runners.) To increase muscle strength without hypertrophy, athletes need to lift very heavy weights using only a few repetitions. Given the intensity and stress of this type of strength training, athletes should spend a few weeks preparing their muscles by first performing a muscular conditioning phase using circuit training, followed by a muscular endurance phase of more formal weight training, using lighter weights with more repetitions.

Plyometric training includes jumping and bounding exercises involving repeated rapid eccentric (lengthening) and concentric (shortening) muscle contractions to improve muscle power. During the stretch-shortening cycle of muscle contraction, muscles produce more force during the concentric contraction if the contraction is immediately preceded by an eccentric contraction. This happens because muscles store elastic energy during the eccentric contraction, which is then used during the subsequent concentric contraction. Plyometric exercises exploit this elastic property of muscles, making the muscles more explosive and powerful. Since a runner's foot is in contact with the ground for only a fraction of a second when racing, there is not enough time to produce maximum force. What's important is the muscles' rate of force production—producing as much force as they can against the ground as quickly as possible. Power equals force times velocity, which can also be thought of as strength times speed. For a muscle to be powerful, it must be strong, and it must be fast.

When doing supplemental training, remember that runners are runners first—never sacrifice running training for supplemental training.

Workout #64: Flexibility Training

Objective: To increase athletes' functional range of motion.

Description: Athletes should perform these active-isolated stretching exercises either after running or apart from their running workouts. A rope can be used to assist at the end of each movement to increase the limb's range of motion.

Coaching Point: For each exercise, athletes should move actively through the range of motion, remembering to contract the muscle group opposing the one being stretched, and use the rope only for light assistance at the end of the range of motion.

Glutes

The athlete should lie on his back and bend the exercising knee, placing the hands behind his knee/thigh (Figure 64-1). Using the abdominals and hip flexors, the athlete lifts the exercising leg toward the chest until he can go no farther. The athlete should gently assist the leg at the end of the stretch with his hands (Figure 64-2). He should hold the stretch for 1 to 2 seconds, return to the starting position, and repeat.

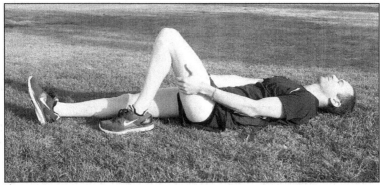

Figure 64-1

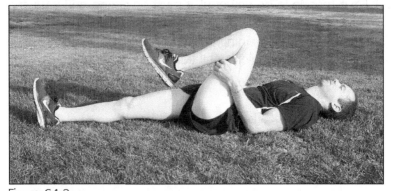

Figure 64-2

Bent-Leg Hamstring

The athlete should lie on his back with both knees bent and feet flat on the ground. The athlete should make a loop with the rope and place the foot of the leg he's exercising into the loop. The athlete should lift his leg until his thigh is perpendicular to the ground (Figure 64-3). He should grasp the ends of the rope with one hand and place the other on top of the thigh of the exercising leg to stabilize it. He should gradually extend the leg by contracting the quadriceps, causing the foot to rise to the ceiling (Figure 64-4). The goal is to lock the knee and have the foot pointing straight up. The athlete should use the rope for gentle assistance at the end of the stretch, but not pull the leg into position. He should hold the stretch for 1 to 2 seconds, return to the starting position, and repeat.

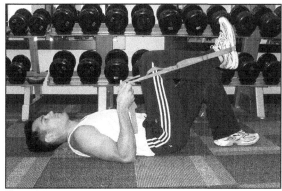
Figure 64-3

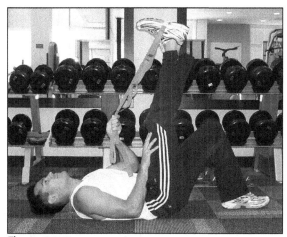
Figure 64-4

Straight-Leg Hamstring

The athlete should lie on his back. He should begin with his non-exercising knee bent and with that foot flat on the ground. The athlete should make a loop with the rope and place the foot of the leg he's exercising into the loop, locking the knee so the leg is extended straight out (Figure 64-5). From the hip and using the quadriceps, he should lift his leg toward his chest, aiming the foot toward the ceiling or sky. He should grasp the ends of the rope with both hands and slightly pull the rope toward him to assist at the end of the stretch, but not pull the leg into position (Figure 64-6). He should hold the stretch for 1 to 2 seconds, return to the starting position, and repeat.

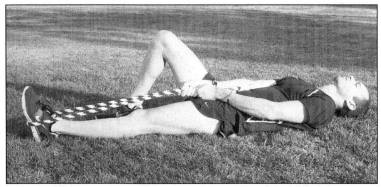

Figure 64-5

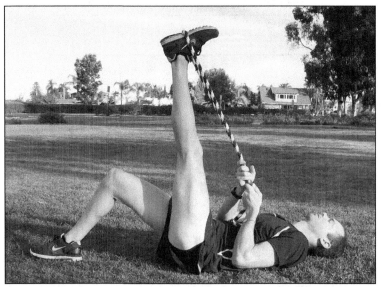

Figure 64-6

Quadriceps

The athlete should lie on her side with her knees bent (in a fetal position). She should slide her bottom arm under the thigh of her bottom leg (Figure 64-7). She should reach down with her upper hand and grasp the shin, ankle, or forefoot of her upper leg. She should keep her knee bent and her leg parallel to the ground. The runner should contract her hamstrings and gluteus maximus, and move the upper leg back as far as she can, using her hand or the rope to give a gentle assist at the end of the stretch (Figure 64-8). She should hold the stretch for 1 to 2 seconds, return to the starting position, and repeat.

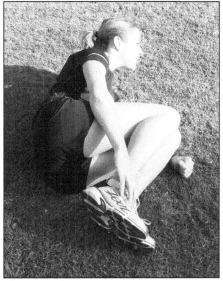

Figure 64-7

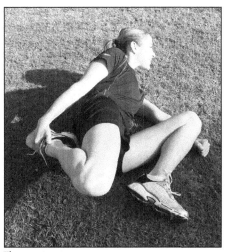

Figure 64-8

Adductors

The athlete should lie on his back with both legs extended straight out, looping the rope around the inside of the ankle, then under the foot, of the exercising leg, so the ends of the rope are on the outside. He should lock that knee and slightly rotate the other leg inward (Figure 64-9). From the hip and using the abductors, the runner should extend the exercising leg out from the side of his body, leading with the heel (Figure 64-10). He should keep slight tension on the rope and use it for gentle assistance at the end of the stretch, but not pull the leg into position. He should hold the stretch for 1 to 2 seconds, return to the starting position, and repeat.

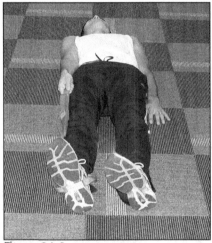

Figure 64-9

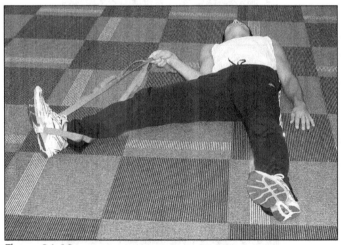

Figure 64-10

Calves

The athlete should sit with both legs straight out in front of him. He should loop a rope around the foot of his exercising leg (Figure 64-11). The runner should flex his foot back toward the ankle, using the rope for a gentle assist at the end of the movement (Figure 64-12). He should hold the stretch for 1 to 2 seconds, return to the starting position, and repeat.

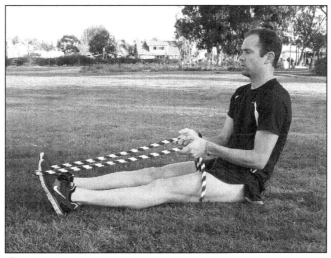

Figure 64-11

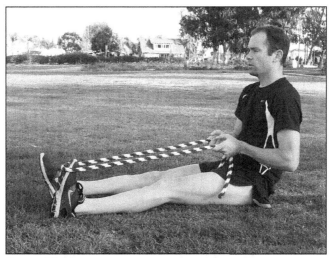

Figure 64-12

Workout #65: Cross Country Running Form Drills

Objective: To improve running form and work on correct running mechanics.

Description: When performing the following drills, athletes should take full recovery between sets to ensure the maintenance of proper form and avoid neuromuscular fatigue.

Coaching Points:
- Always watch drills so you can help athletes to "mold" the drill to perfection. It's better to not do the drills at all than to do them with improper form, since that will only create and ingrain bad habits.
- For all of these drills, athletes should remain either on the midfoot or the ball of the foot. These drills are great for training young runners who are severe heel-strikers.

High-Knee Walk

This drill focuses on the hip flexors. The athlete should march two to four sets of 30 meters, bringing the hip to 90 degrees so that the thighs are parallel to the ground. He should focus on creating 90-degree angles at the knee and at the ankle. Legs should come down directly underneath his center of gravity and land on the midfoot (Figure 65-1).

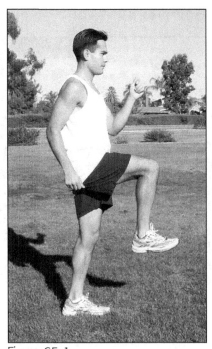

Figure 65-1

High-Knee Skip

This drill is similar to the high-knee walk, but is performed as a skip, focusing on three 90-degree angles: hip, knee, and ankle (Figure 65-2). The runner should do two to four sets of 30 meters.

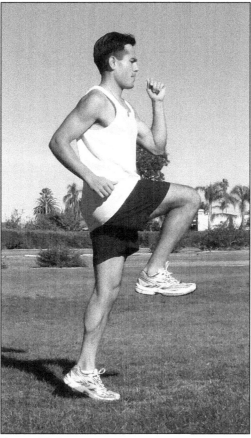

Figure 65-2

High-Knee Run

This drill is similar to the high-knee walk and skip, but is performed as a run. The horizontal distance is covered slowly, as the emphasis is on moving the legs up and down as fast as possible, like a piston or sewing machine. The athlete should think of the ground as hot coals, picking the leg up as soon as it touches the ground. He should remain on the ball of his foot (Figure 65-3). The runner should do two to four sets of 30 meters.

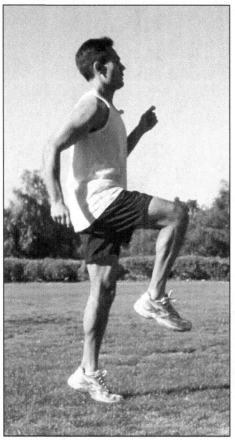

Figure 65-3

Butt Kicks

This drill focuses on the hamstrings. The athlete should run two to four sets of 30 meters, focusing on flexing the knees and flicking the back of the butt with the heels of the shoes. Emphasis is on moving the legs quickly (Figure 65-4). The runner should do two to four sets of 30 meters.

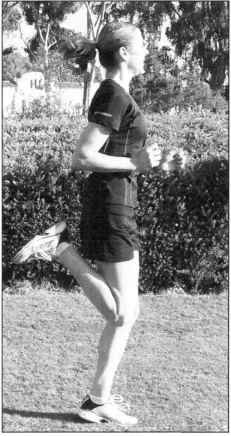

Figure 65-4

Running Leg Cycle

All of the previously outlined drills come into play in this drill, which takes athletes' legs through the entire running cycle. The athlete should lean against a fence or pole and, while standing in place, move his leg through the entire running cycle—starting with the foot on the ground (Figure 65-5), extending the leg at the hip and sweeping the leg back (Figure 65-6), bending the knee and pulling the knee to the front of his body until the hip is at 90 degrees (also creating 90-degree angles at the knee and ankle) (Figure 65-7), then lowering the leg to the ground under his center of gravity, and repeating. He should think, "Land, push off, pull through; land, push off, pull through." The runner should do two to three sets of 20 reps with each leg.

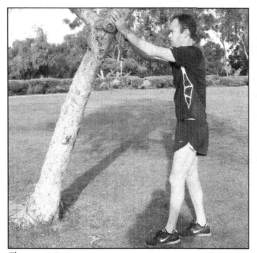
Figure 65-5

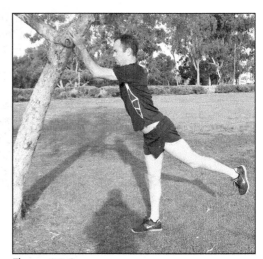
Figure 65-6

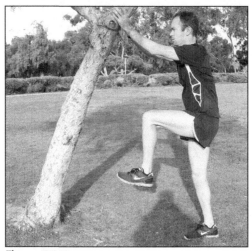
Figure 65-7

Bounding

In an exaggerated running motion, the athlete should bound (which looks like a combination of running and jumping) forward from one leg to the other (Figure 65-8). He should do two to four sets of 40 to 50 meters.

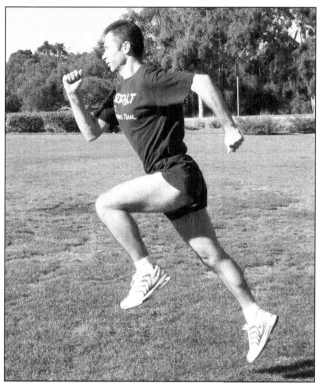

Figure 65-8

Workout #66: Core Circuit

Objective: To improve strength and endurance of the core muscles as part of the athlete's supplemental training.

Description: Athletes should do the circuit two to three times and do each exercise for 30 seconds, moving from one exercise to the next with no rest in between.

Coaching Point: Ensure that athletes use proper form for each exercise.

Traditional Crunch

The athlete should lie on his back on the ground, lift his legs, bend his knees, and cross his feet at the ankles. He should place his hands across his chest or behind his head (Figure 66-1). He should contract the abs, lifting the shoulder blades and upper back off the ground (Figure 66-2). He can add resistance by holding a medicine ball against his chest or by lying on a decline bench and raising his torso against gravity.

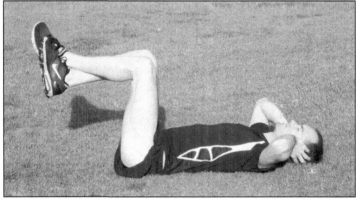

Figure 66-1

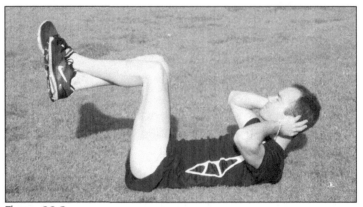

Figure 66-2

Push-Ups

The athlete should kneel on the ground with his hands slightly less than shoulder-width apart and palms on the ground, legs lifted off the ground, and back straight and parallel to the ground (Figure 66-3). He should lower himself down until his chest touches the ground (Figure 66-4). He should push himself back up until his arms are straight, and repeat. Female athletes can modify this standard push-up position by placing the knees on the ground and flexed to 90 degrees with the ankles crossed (Figures 66-5 and 66-6). To make the abs work while doing push-ups, the athlete should place the hands on a stability ball instead of on the ground.

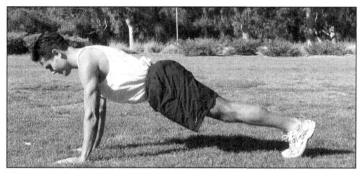

Figure 66-3

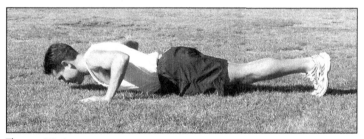

Figure 66-4

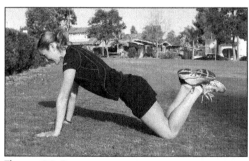

Figure 66-5

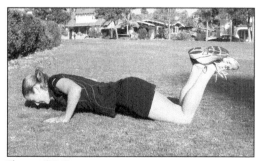

Figure 66-6

Reverse Crunch

The athlete should lie on his back on the ground and hold onto a teammate's ankles above his head. He should raise his legs up and back toward his teammate (Figure 66-7). He should have his teammate grab his feet and toss them down and in different directions. The athlete should squeeze his abs to prevent his legs from falling to the ground and "pull" his legs back to his teammate (Figure 66-8). He should keep his back flat against the ground.

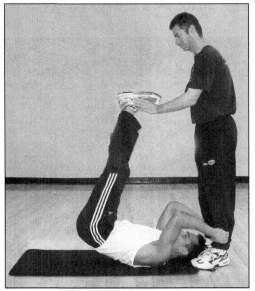

Figure 66-7

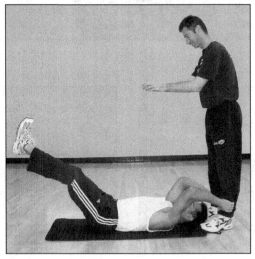

Figure 66-8

Superman

The athlete should lie face down on the ground, with legs together and straight, and arms straight and extended above his head. He should keep his head and neck in a neutral position (Figure 66-9). Keeping his torso stationary, he should lift his right arm and left leg about 5 to 6 inches off the ground (Figure 66-10). He should lower those limbs while raising the left arm and right leg.

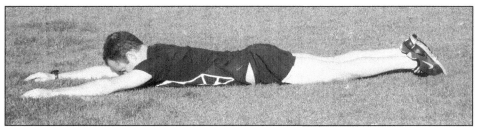

Figure 66-9

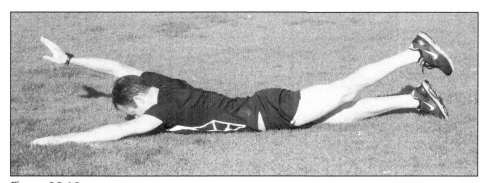

Figure 66-10

Medicine-Ball Crunch

The athlete should lie on his back on the ground, bend his knees, and place his feet flat on the ground. With a teammate standing in front of him, he should have the teammate throw him a medicine ball in different directions—straight at him, to the left, and to the right (Figure 66-11). The athlete should catch the ball by moving only his torso and arms, do a crunch with the medicine ball, and throw the medicine ball back to his teammate (Figure 66-12). He can add resistance by increasing the weight of the medicine ball.

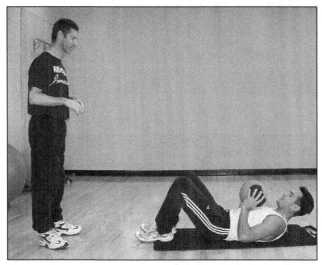

Figure 66-11

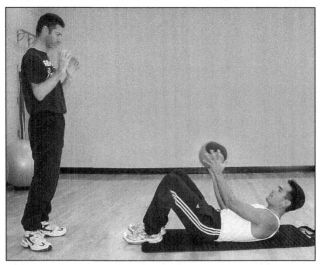

Figure 66-12

Side Plank

The athlete should lie on her side with her right hand or elbow and forearm on the ground (Figure 66-13). She should lift herself up to form a plank with her right arm straight (or bent at the elbow) and her left arm on her side or pointing up in the air (Figure 66-14). She should repeat with the other side, and keep her body in a straight line.

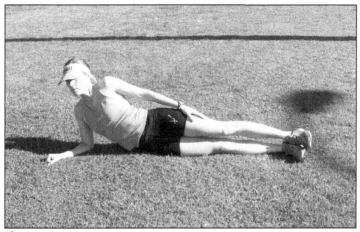

Figure 66-13

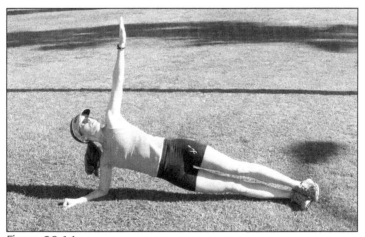

Figure 66-14

V-Sit

The athlete should lie on his back on the ground with knees bent at 90 degrees and hips flexed at about 45 degrees. He should keep his arms to the sides with the palms of his hands on the ground (Figure 66-15). He should contract the abs and curl the upper body while simultaneously bringing his knees toward his chest to create a V shape. The hips should be the point of the V as he balances on his buttocks in the V position (Figure 66-16).

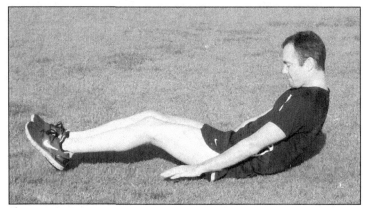

Figure 66-15

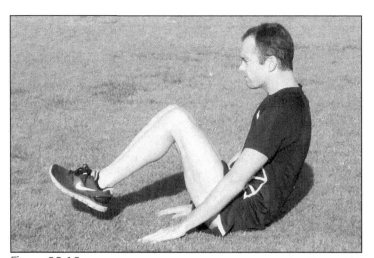

Figure 66-16

Workout #67: Power Circuit

Objective: To increase muscle power using dumbbells and body-weight exercises as part of the athlete's supplemental training.

Description: This non-stop circuit pairs a dumbbell exercise with an explosive plyometric exercise using the athlete's body weight.

Coaching Points:
- Athletes should do the circuit two to three times and do each exercise for 30 seconds, moving from one exercise to the next with no rest in between. Rest 5 minutes between sets.
- For each dumbbell exercise, athletes should use a weight that will almost fully fatigue their muscles in 30 seconds.
- Athletes should do plyometric exercises on a soft surface.

Rotated Chest Press

With one dumbbell gripped in each hand, the athlete should lie on his back on a bench. Feet should touch the ground with knees bent at 90 degrees. He should begin with elbows bent at 90 degrees and the palms of his hands facing toward him (Figure 67-1). In one curved motion, he should straighten his arms and bring the dumbbells in toward the midline of the chest while rotating his hands so his palms face away from him until the ends of the dumbbells meet. Elbows should remain slightly bent at the top of the movement (Figure 67-2). He should lower the dumbbells back down to the starting position, and repeat.

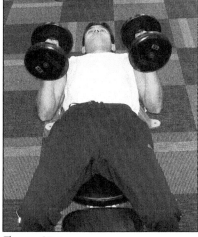

Figure 67-1

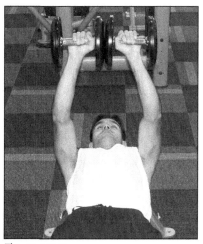

Figure 67-2

Power Push-Ups

The athlete should get into a push-up position, with his back straight and hands shoulder-width apart on the edge of the bench. He should lower himself down until his chest comes close to the bench (Figure 67-3). He should straighten his arms to push himself up (Figure 67-4), letting go of the bench at the end of the movement (Figure 67-5). He should catch himself on the bench, and repeat.

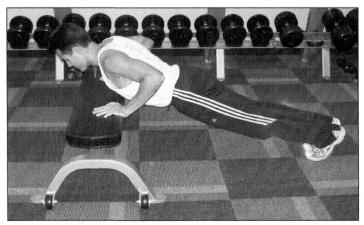

Figure 67-3

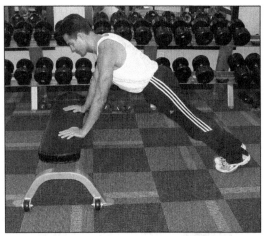

Figure 67-4

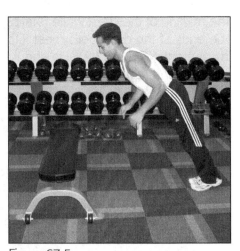

Figure 67-5

Bench Squats

The athlete should stand in front of a bench with his right leg bent and resting on the bench (Figure 67-6). He should bend his left knee and lower himself straight down to do a one-legged squat (Figure 67-7). He should make sure his squatting leg does not rotate inward. He should squat with each leg for 15 seconds.

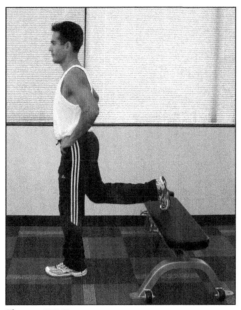

Figure 67-6

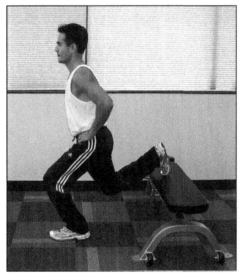

Figure 67-7

Squat Jumps

The athlete should begin in a squat position with his thighs parallel to the ground and hands on his hips (Figure 67-8). He should jump straight up as high as possible (Figure 67-9). He should land with soft knees, lowering himself back into a squat position in one smooth motion, and immediately jump up again.

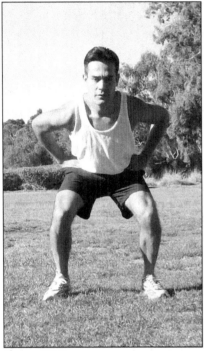

Figure 67-8

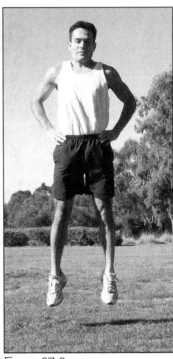

Figure 67-9

Renegades

The athlete should place dumbbells vertically on the ground. He should stand over the dumbbells, with legs shoulder-width apart and bent at the waist. He should grab the dumbbells with palms facing each other (Figure 67-10). He should do an alternating row, quickly pulling one dumbbell at a time toward his chest by bending elbow (Figure 67-11). He should lower each arm back down, and repeat.

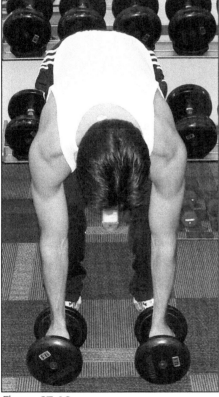
Figure 67-10

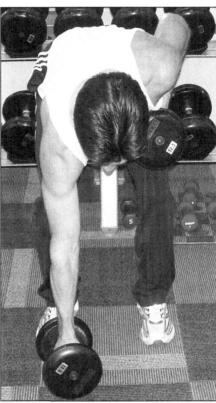
Figure 67-11

Medicine-Ball Toss

The athlete should stand with his feet shoulder-width apart. With knees slightly bent and abdominals tight, he should throw an 8- to 10-pound medicine ball with two hands from his chest straight up into the air like a volleyball pass (Figure 67-12). He should catch the medicine ball with outstretched arms, drawing his arms into his chest in one smooth movement, and quickly throw it back up again (Figure 67-13). This exercise can also be done by throwing the medicine ball back and forth to a teammate.

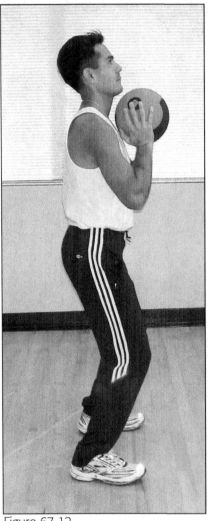
Figure 67-12

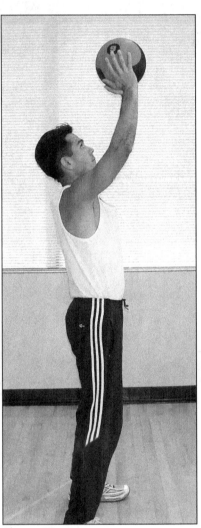
Figure 67-13

Fencer's Lunge

The athlete should stand with her legs shoulder-width apart. She should turn her right leg 90 degrees to her right and turn her body so that she is facing to her right (Figure 67-14). She should lunge her right leg forward like a fencer, keeping her back straight, chest out, and shoulders back. She should keep her back leg straight (Figure 67-15). She should push off with her right heel to the starting position. She should lunge with each leg for 15 seconds.

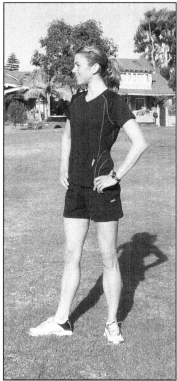

Figure 67-14

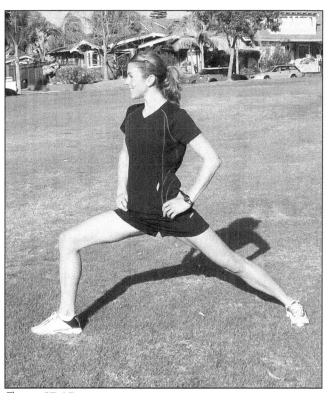

Figure 67-15

Split-Jump Lunges

From a forward lunge position (a squat with one leg in front of the other) (Figure 67-16), the athlete should jump up while switching leg position in mid-air (Figure 67-17). She should land with soft knees, lowering back down into a lunge position (Figure 67-18).

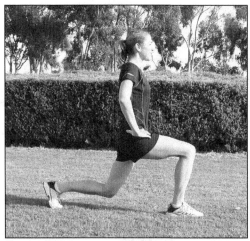
Figure 67-16

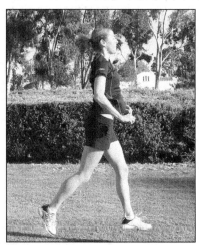
Figure 67-17

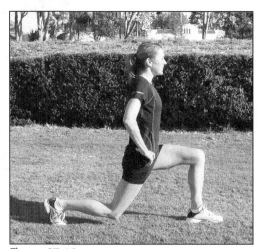
Figure 67-18

Workout #68: Running Circuit

Objective: To condition the athletes and prepare them for more formal training.

Description: This workout integrates periods of running with body-weight exercises performed during the recovery intervals. Athletes should do the circuit two to three times.

- 400-meter run
- 20 squat jumps
- 20 crunches
- 20 push-ups
- 400-meter run
- 20 forward lunges (Figure 68-1)

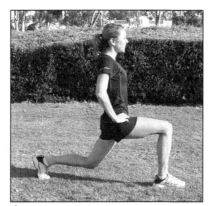

Figure 68-1

- Sprint/backpedal drill (Figure 68-2): The athlete should sprint to the first cone, change direction quickly, backpedal to the next cone, and repeat the sequence.

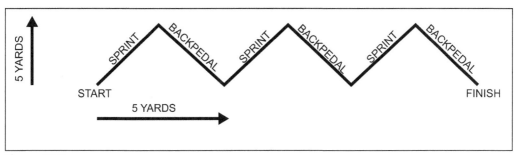

Figure 68-2

- 20 V-sits
- 400-meter run
- 20 overhead presses (with resistance band or dumbbells): The athlete should stand with his feet shoulder-width apart. He should hold a dumbbell (or the handles of a resistance band) in each hand with elbows bent and pointing down and palms facing forward (Figures 68-3 and 68-5). He should press the dumbbells (or resistance band handles) up and in together over his head until they meet (Figures 68-4 and 68-6). He should then lower the dumbbells (or resistance band handles), keeping the resistance balanced over his elbows until the elbows are just below shoulder-level.
- 20 crunches
- 20 push-ups

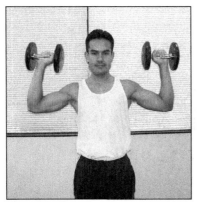
Figure 68-3

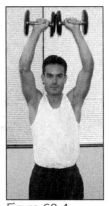
Figure 68-4

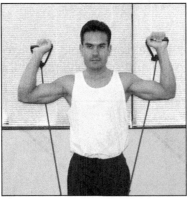
Figure 68-5

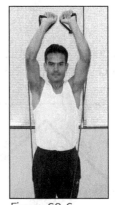
Figure 68-6

Coaching Points:
- The running periods should be challenging, but the exact pace is not important.
- The workout should be fatiguing enough that it improves the conditioning of the athlete, but not so fatiguing that it takes away from the other running-specific workouts.

Workout #69: Muscular Endurance

Objective: To increase muscle endurance as part of the athlete's supplemental training and prepare the athlete's muscles for the subsequent muscular strength training.

Description: Athletes should do two to three sets of 15 to 20 reps at 70 percent of their one-rep max (the maximum amount of weight that can be lifted just once) with 30 to 60 seconds rest between sets.

Coaching Points:
- A training cycle of muscular endurance workouts should precede the muscular strength workouts.
- If it is impractical to test each athlete's one-rep max for each exercise, have the athletes choose a weight that will fatigue their muscles within the prescribed rep range.

UPPER BODY

Bench Press

The athlete should lie on his back on a flat bench with his feet flat on the floor and his chest directly underneath the barbell. He should grip the barbell with an overhand grip and hands greater than shoulder-width apart (Figure 69-1). He should lift the barbell from the rack and lower the weight to his chest (Figure 69-2). He should push the barbell back up to the starting position until his arms are fully extended, and repeat.

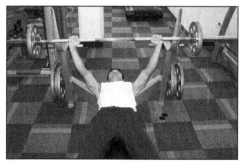
Figure 69-1

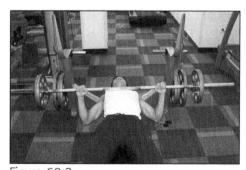
Figure 69-2

Seated Row

The athlete should sit on the seat of the seated row machine, with her back straight and her feet flat on the foot rests. She should grab the handles (Figure 69-3). She should use her back muscles to pull the handles to her chest (Figure 69-4). She should extend her arms to lower the weight back to the starting position.

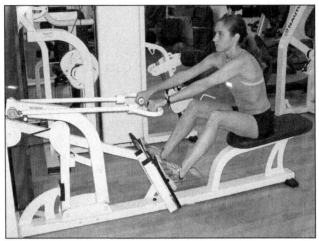

Figure 69-3

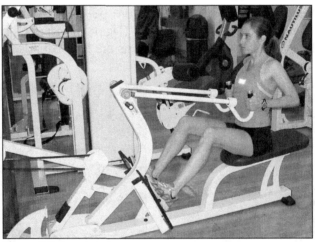

Figure 69-4

Chin-Ups

The athlete should grab a horizontal chin-up bar or the handles of a jungle gym with an underhand grip (palms facing him) and his hands shoulder-width apart (Figure 69-5). From a hanging position with legs either straight or bent at the knees, he should pull his body up until his chin is above the bar (Figure 69-6). He should not swing his body. He should lower his body until his arms are fully extended, and repeat. He can also do pull-ups instead of chin-ups by grabbing the bar or handles with an overhand grip (palms facing away from him). To make the exercise more difficult, he should use a wide grip. If an athlete cannot lift his body weight, he can use a weight-assisted chin-up machine like the Gravitron®, which allows the athlete to stand on a platform or a bar with a counterweight to reduce the weight that he pulls up.

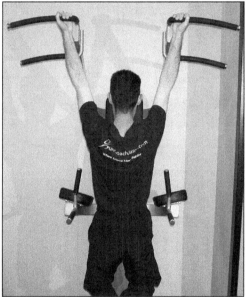

Figure 69-5

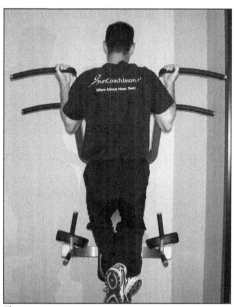

Figure 69-6

Push-Ups

The athlete should kneel on the ground with hands slightly less than shoulder-width apart and palms on the ground, legs lifted off the ground, and back straight and parallel to the ground (Figure 69-7). He should lower himself down until his chest touches the ground (Figure 69-8). He should push himself back up until his arms are straight, and repeat. Female athletes can modify this standard push-up position by placing knees on the ground and flexed to 90 degrees with ankles crossed (Figures 69-9 and 69-10). To make the abs work while doing push-ups, the athlete can place the hands on a stability ball instead of on the ground.

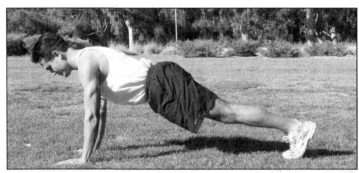

Figure 69-7

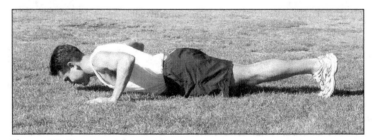

Figure 69-8

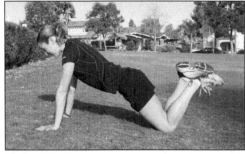

Figure 69-9

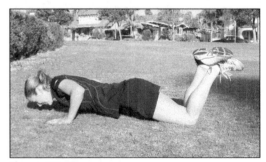

Figure 69-10

Cable Crossovers

With the pulley set down by his feet, the athlete should stand with his feet shoulder-width apart next to the pulley. He should bend down to grab the pulley across his body with an overhand grip. He should stand up while holding the pulley. His hand should touch his opposite hip (Figure 69-11). He should use his upper back muscles to lift his arm up and away from his body until his arm is fully extended (Figure 69-12). He should then lower his arm back down across his body to return the weight to the starting position.

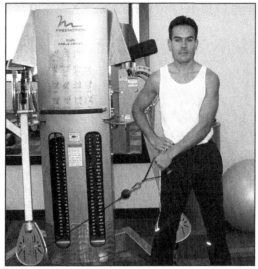

Figure 69-11

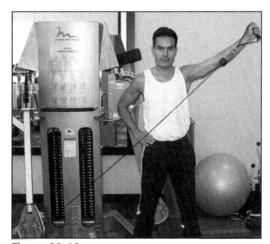

Figure 69-12

LOWER BODY

Leg Press

The athlete should sit on a leg-press machine with his feet shoulder-width apart on the platform and his back flat against the back pad. He should adjust the seat position so that his knees are bent at 90 degrees. He should grasp the side handles for support (Figure 69-13). He should lift the weight by pressing his feet against the platform and straightening his legs until just before the legs are straight (he shouldn't lock the knees) (Figure 69-14). Throughout the motion, he should keep his legs parallel to one another. He should bend his knees to lower the weight back down to the starting position.

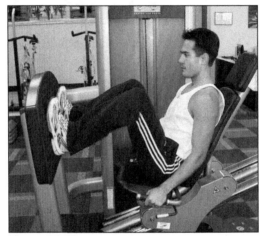

Figure 69-13

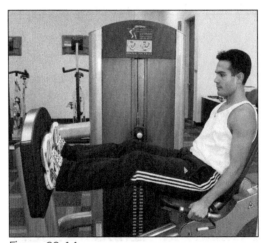

Figure 69-14

Squats

With his feet shoulder-width or slightly greater than shoulder-width apart, the athlete should stand in front of a barbell that is sitting on a rack. He should place the barbell across the back of his shoulders below the neck and grab the barbell from behind with a grip slightly greater than shoulder-width. He should lift the barbell off the rack so it rests on his shoulders and upper back (Figure 69-15). Keeping the back straight, he should bend his knees and squat down until his thighs are parallel to the floor. He should move his hips back as if attempting to sit in a chair (Figure 69-16). He should straighten his legs and stand up to return to the starting position.

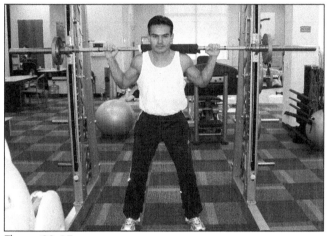

Figure 69-15

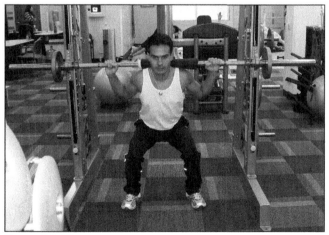

Figure 69-16

Power Cleans

The athlete should stand with his feet hip- to shoulder-width apart. He should bend his legs and grab a barbell with an overhand grip at slightly wider than shoulder-width. Thighs should be parallel to the floor, with shoulders square and directly over the bar (Figure 69-17). To lift the barbell, he should push with his legs, keeping his back straight. When the bar passes the knees, he should bend the legs again to lower his upper body so his chest passes underneath the bar (Figure 69-18). He should push his legs to a standing position, with the bar resting in front of his shoulders (Figure 69-19). From the standing position, he should bend the legs again and drop his arms to lower the bar back to the starting position.

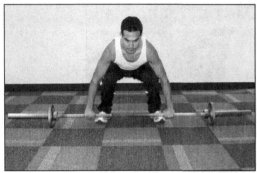
Figure 69-17

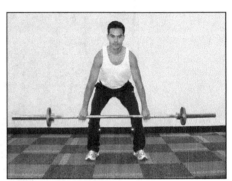
Figure 69-18

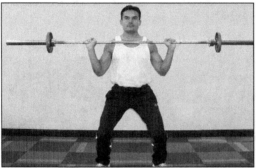
Figure 69-19

Hamstring Curls

The athlete should lie on his stomach on the floor with a resistance band looped around his ankle and tethered to an immovable object (Figure 69-20). He should curl his leg toward his butt (Figure 69-21). The athlete can also use a hamstring curl machine with the pad just below the calves and the hips flat against the bench, adjusting position so that the knees are in line with the pivot point of the machine (Figures 69-22 and 69-23).

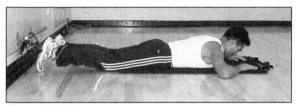

Figure 69-20

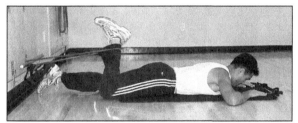

Figure 69-21

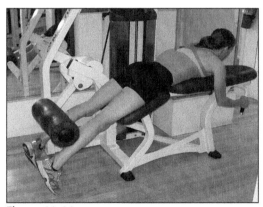

Figure 69-22

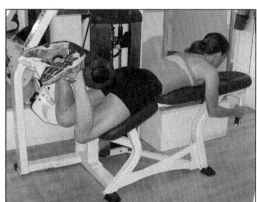

Figure 69-23

Calf Raises

The athlete should stand with the feet together, with one foot off the ground (Figure 69-24). With the other foot, she should push against the ground with the ball of her foot to raise herself up (Figure 69-25). To make the exercise more difficult, she can hold a dumbbell in each hand or rest a barbell or weighted bar across the back of her shoulders and neck. She can also do calf raises on the edge of a stair or platform by hanging her heel over the edge (Figures 69-26 and 69-27).

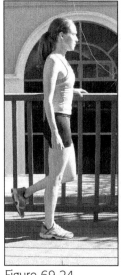
Figure 69-24

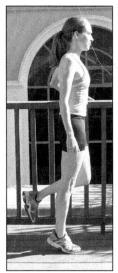
Figure 69-25

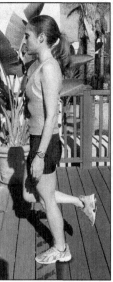
Figure 69-26

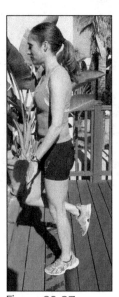
Figure 69-27

Workout #70: Muscular Strength

Objective: To increase muscle strength as part of the athlete's supplemental training and prepare the athlete's muscles and tendons for the subsequent muscular power training.

Description: Athletes should do three to four sets of three to five reps at 90 percent of their one-rep max with 5 minutes rest between sets. All of the exercises described for Workout #69: Muscular Endurance can be used.

Coaching Points:
- While it may be beneficial for some younger athletes to increase muscle mass, this workout should be done using near-maximal weights and only a few reps per set so that strength is increased via a neural, rather than hypertrophic (muscle growth), mechanism so as not to increase muscle size, which would have a negative impact on running economy.
- If it is impractical to test each athlete's one-rep max for each exercise, have the athletes choose a weight that will fatigue their muscles within the prescribed rep range.
- Make sure athletes maintain proper form when doing strength training exercises.

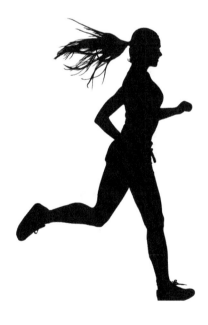

Workout #71: Plyometrics

Objective: To increase muscle power as part of the athlete's supplemental training.

Description: Athletes should begin with two sets of 10 reps of each exercise, progressing to four sets, with full recovery between sets.

Coaching Points:
- Plyometric exercises should always be performed on soft surfaces with good footing, such as grass, artificial turf, or wrestling mat.
- Precede a plyometric workout with a general warm-up that gradually gets more intense.
- Athletes should concentrically contract their muscles immediately after eccentrically contracting them by trying to spend as little time on the ground as possible between hops, bounds, and jumps.
- High-intensity plyometric exercises, such as depth jumps and box jumps, should be included in the athlete's program only after mastery of lower-intensity and moderate-intensity exercises (e.g., single-leg hops, leg bounds, and squat jumps).

Single-Leg Hops

On a grass field or other soft surface, the athlete should do three hopping exercises on one leg at a time: hop up and down (Figures 71-1 and 71-2), hop forward and back (Figures 71-3 and 71-4), and hop from side to side (Figures 71-5 and 71-6). The focus of these hops is the ankle joint, with the power coming from the gastrocnemius muscle in the calf.

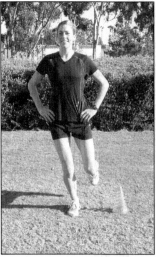
Figure 71-1

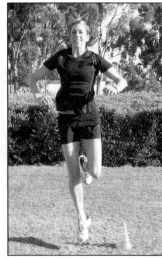
Figure 71-2

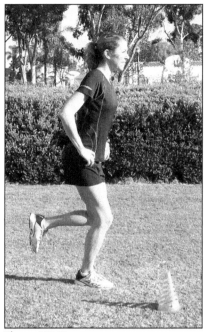

Figure 71-3

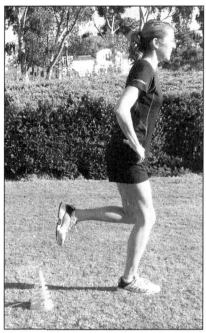

Figure 71-4

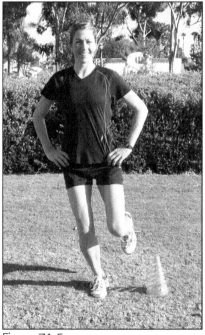

Figure 71-5

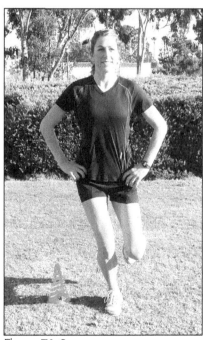

Figure 71-6

Double-Leg Bound

The athlete should bend her legs in a squat position with her thighs parallel to the ground (Figure 71-7). She should jump forward with both legs as far as possible (Figure 71-8) and land in a squat position (Figure 71-9).

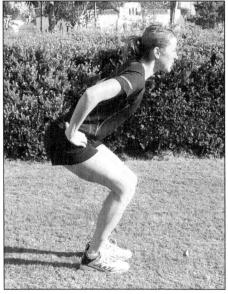

Figure 71-7

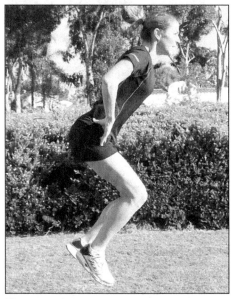

Figure 71-8

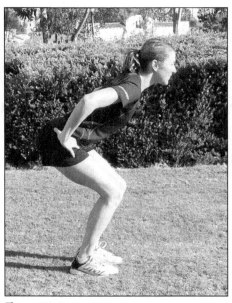

Figure 71-9

Squat Jumps

The athlete should begin with hands on his hips in a squat position (Figure 71-10). He should jump straight up as high as possible (Figure 71-11). Upon landing with soft knees, he should lower back into a squat position in one smooth motion, and immediately jump up again.

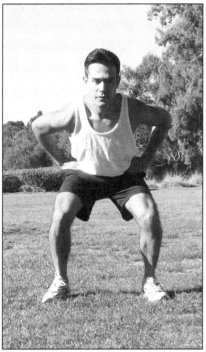

Figure 71-10

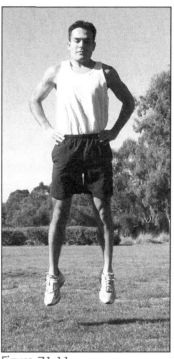

Figure 71-11

Depth Jumps

From a standing position on a two-foot-tall box (Figure 71-12), the athlete should jump onto the ground and land in a squat position (Figure 71-13). From this squat position, she should jump straight up as high as possible (Figure 71-14).

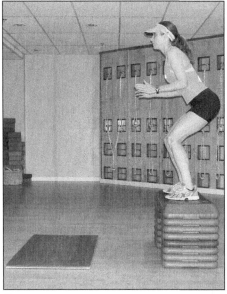

Figure 71-12

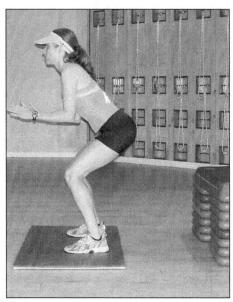

Figure 71-13

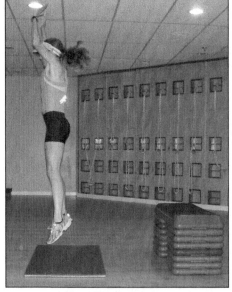

Figure 71-14

Box Jumps

The athlete should stand with feet shoulder-width apart and knees bent in a squat position in front of a box about two feet high (Figure 71-15). She should jump with two feet onto the box (Figure 71-16). She should immediately jump into the air and back down to the ground on the other side of the box, landing in a squat position (Figure 71-17). As she gets experienced with the exercise, she can try jumping with one foot at a time.

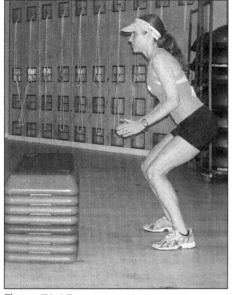

Figure 71-15

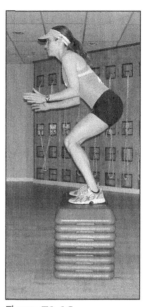

Figure 71-16

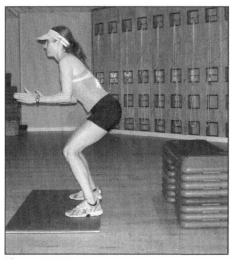

Figure 71-17

About the Author

Jason Karp, Ph.D., is owner of RunCoachJason.com, a coaching, personal training, and consulting company, offering science-based coaching to runners of all levels, fitness training to the public, and consulting to coaches and runners. He is a frequent presenter at national fitness, coaching, and academic conferences. He has taught USA Track & Field's highest level coaching certification and was an instructor at the USATF/U.S. Olympic Committee's Emerging Elite Coaching Camp at the U.S. Olympic Training Center. He is also the founder and host of the $\dot{V}O_2$max Distance Running Clinic for runners, coaches, and fitness professionals; the San Diego Personal Training Summit for personal trainers; Dr. Karp's Run-Fit Boot Camp; and Running Clinics & Workouts in the Park™, a series of running clinics and workouts for runners of all abilities. He is a prolific writer, with over 100 articles published in numerous international coaching, running, and fitness trade and consumer magazines, including *Track Coach*, *Techniques for Track & Field and Cross Country*, *New Studies in Athletics*, *Running Times*, *Runner's World*, *Trail Runner*, *Marathon & Beyond*, *IDEA Fitness Journal*, *PTontheNet.com*, *Shape*, *Oxygen*, *SELF*, *Ultra-Fit*, and *Maximum Fitness*, among others. He is also author of *How to Survive Your PhD* (Sourcebooks, 2009) and the forthcoming *Women's Running Bible* (Human Kinetics, 2012).

In 1997, at the age of 24, Karp became one of the youngest head college coaches in the country, leading the Georgian Court University (NJ) women's cross country team to the regional championship and was named NAIA Northeast Region Coach of the Year. During that time, he was also a personal trainer and a hospital fitness specialist. After moving to San Francisco, he coached two high school teams, helping a few athletes to win city championship titles and qualify for the state championships. He also coached the elite women's Impala Racing Team and recreational marathon runners for San Francisco Fit®. As a private coach and founder of *REVO₂LT Running Team*™, he has helped many runners meet their potential, ranging from a first-time race participant to an Olympic Trials qualifier. A competitive runner himself, Karp is a USA Track & Field certified coach and is sponsored by PowerBar® as a member of PowerBar Team Elite™.

Karp received his Ph.D. in exercise physiology with a physiology minor from Indiana University in 2007, his master's degree in kinesiology from the University of Calgary in 1997, and his bachelor's degree in exercise and sport science with an English minor from Pennsylvania State University in 1995. His research has included motor-unit recruitment during eccentric muscle contractions, post-exercise nutrition for optimal recovery in endurance athletes, training characteristics of Olympic marathon trials qualifiers, and the coordination of breathing and stride rate in highly trained distance runners. His research has been published in the scientific journals *Medicine and Science in Sports and Exercise*, *International Journal of Sport Nutrition and Exercise Metabolism*, and *International Journal of Sports Physiology and Performance*. Karp has taught exercise physiology and biomechanics at several universities, and he has taught in the fitness certificate program at the University of California at Berkeley. He is adjunct faculty at Miramar College in San Diego, where he teaches applied exercise physiology.